Defeat Neuropathy – Now!

Inspite of Your Doctor

Dr. John Coppola D.C.
Dr. Valerie Monteiro D.C.

Neuropathydoctorsa.com

Copyright 2012 by Dr. John Coppola, DC and Dr. Valerie Monteiro, DC

No part of this publication may be reproduced by any mechanical, photographic, or electronic process, or in the form of a phonographic or audio recording; nor may it be stored in a retrieval system, transmitted in any form or by any means, electronic, mechanical, photocopying, recording, scanning, or otherwise, except as permitted under Section 107 or 108 of the 1976 United States Copyright Act, without the prior written permission of the publisher. Nor can it be copied for public or private use—other than for "fair use" as brief quotations embodied in articles and reviews—without prior written permission of the publisher.

Defeat Neuropathy Now!

ISBN: 1482084538
ISBN-13: 9781482084535

Author: Dr. John Coppola, DC and Dr. Valerie Monteiro, DC

LIMITS OF LIABILITY / DISCLAIMER OF WARRANTY: The content of this book is provided for information purposes only. The content is intended to provide you with information only and not replace the advice and counsel of a doctor nor constitute a doctor-patient relationship. Never disregard medical advice or delay seeking treatment because of information that you have read in this book. The information presented is not to be considered complete, nor does it contain all medical resource information that may be relevant, and therefore is not intended as a substitute for seeking appropriate care.

All content, including text, graphics, images, and information available in this book, is for educational purposes only and is not sufficient for medical decisions. The content is not intended to be a substitute for professional medical advice, diagnosis, or treatment.

By using this book, you agree to hold harmless and shall not seek remedy from John Coppola, DC and Valerie Monteiro, DC. The authors and publisher disclaim all liability to you for damages, costs, and expenses, including legal fees because of your reliance on anything derived from this book, and furthermore assume no liability for any and all claims arising out of the said use, regardless of the cause, effects, or fault.

First Printing, 2013

Printed in the United States of America

Neuropathydoctorsa.com

In Loving Memory of Jenny Monteiro...

My Hero

DEDICATION

We dedicate this book to all of our patients, including the ones we have not met yet. Through working with all of you, we have learned more than we ever did in school. We thank you for taking the final leap of faith with us and for allowing us to be part of your journey in healing.

We promise to do our very best to pour as much effort into your health as you have poured into us.

Yours in health,

Dr. Coppola and Dr. Monteiro

TABLE OF CONTENTS

Acknowledgement ix
Foreword xi
Preface xiii
Introduction xv
Patient Testimonials. xix
1. The Great Neuropathy Hoax 1
2. Lies Your Drug Company Doesn't Want You to Know About. 15
3. Freedom From Peripheral Neuropathy 33
4. Shocking Facts About Your Medications and Neuropathy. . 45
5. What Your Doctor Didn't Tell You. 73
6. Proven Treatments to Reverse Neuropathy. 107
7. The Foods You Eat May Be Killing Your Nerves 117
8. Nutrients to Heal Nerves 137
9. Rebuilding Nerves-One Meal at a Time 165
10. Move it and Lose the Neuropathy 217
11. Take Back Control. 227
12. Formulating a Game Plan 235
Glossary 245

ACKNOWLEDGEMENT

We wish to personally thank the following people for their inspiration, support and guidance in helping to create our book.

We would like to give a heartfelt thank you to Dr. Brian Beckner. You provided us with the vision of turning a simple educational pamphlet into a book that we are truly proud of. The feedback you gave us on the manuscript helped us to shape the book. Your advice has been invaluable.

No one walks alone down the pathway of life. It is for this reason that I would like to express my sincere gratitude to a man who guided me along my journey, Dr. Gary Alves. You have been a lifelong mentor. You first hired a young, tenacious girl as your medical assistant and then encouraged her to 'reach for the stars.' Your advice and support throughout my career has been instrumental. We appreciated—immensely—your feedback on the rough draft of this book. It was 'spot on' and helped us to create a better version than the first manuscript.

Lastly, we would like to acknowledge Mike Adams, the Health Crusader. We are incredibly grateful for all the work that you do in educating the public on their health. Your passion pours forth in your work at NaturalNews.com and inspires the likes of us daily. We thank you for your courage and fortitude. We also thank you for sharing your comic medical satire with us. It helps tremendously to take a serious topic and add some levity while still being informative. Please don't ever stop your crusading.

FOREWORD

If you are reading this book, chances are you are currently taking a prescription drug for neuropathy or other conditions. Americans are taking more prescription medications than we've ever seen in the past. Statistics show that one out of two Americans is currently on a prescribed drug now, with a 71 percent increase in prescription purchases, as reported in a study conducted by the Henry J. Kaiser Family Foundation (a nonprofit organization). Regularly, we still encounter patients who are taking multiple medications, often prescribed by different doctors, with significant overlap and duplication in these medications. Unfortunately this leaves us, as a nation, battling numerous adverse effects of polypharmacy.

Drug companies, in their endless greed and pursuit of profit, now push more medications than ever before with the help of the FDA. The pharmaceutical industry spends $57.4 billion on marketing, which is double the amount spent on research and development of a drug. Furthermore, seductive and enticing drug advertising now has patients requesting medications by name from their physicians, based on information acquired from commercials.

In the age of managed health care, physicians are under significant pressure to manage increasing numbers of patients in less time. This leaves little time for the doctor to counsel their patients on necessary lifestyle changes. The result—increased medical prescriptions in an attempt to achieve rapid results.

In addition, in our modern society people want the *fast fix*, while taking little responsibility for their personal health. This is due, in part, to complacency by some patients, but overall it is caused largely by the confusion about where a person suffering from neuropathy should begin in their pursuit of health.

I applaud Dr. Monteiro and Dr. Coppola for writing this groundbreaking book to help dispel the many myths about neuropathy. I admire the fact that they have gone to extensive lengths to provide the reader with the most current research on nerve repair. Even more important, this book provides the reader with a *recovery road map* from neuropathy. What I love about this book is that it arms the patient with appropriate questions to ask their doctor, while educating them on the simple things they can incorporate into their lifestyle. It will give the average person the ability to make important, informed medical decisions when confronted with the diagnosis of neuropathy. This will ultimately aid them in winning the battle against peripheral neuropathy.

This text is extremely informative, yet still maintains a witty and entertaining tone. You don't have to be a scientist to understand the book. It is an easy read for everyone. *Defeat Neuropathy Now!* will most certainly be appreciated by anyone suffering from neuropathy. This is required reading for individuals wanting to take an active role in their health care.

Dr. Jeffrey Swift, DC, DABCN
Diplomate, American Board of Chiropractic Neurologists

PREFACE

WHAT IF EVERYTHING YOU WERE TOLD ABOUT NEUROPATHY WAS WRONG?

If you are reading this book, you are likely suffering from peripheral neuropathy, or you have a loved one who suffers from peripheral neuropathy. In our modern world, neuropathy has become quite prevalent. It is a devastating and debilitating condition. You try your best to understand the disease, but somehow it's elusive. You try to get answers from your doctor, but all you get are medications. All of your hope is crushed as your doctor tells you, "Just learn to live with it."

It's time that you knew the truth. **There is hope, and your nerves can heal and regenerate**! This isn't merely our opinion. This is based on the scientific evidence that has been published. You ask, "Why doesn't my doctor know about this research?" Unfortunately, most doctors, regardless of their specialty, are overwhelmed with the large volume of patient care – leaving them little to no time to stay on top of the current research.

This book is designed to bring you up to speed on the latest groundbreaking research and to debunk old myths about neuropathy. It will help you understand the actual cause of your neuropathy and provide you with the most up-to-date information on what can be done to heal your nerves. This book also includes testimonials from patients who had lost hope while suffering from this condition, only to be astonished to find out that their neuropathy was reversible.

Most important, this book was designed to let you know that ...

YOU DON'T HAVE TO LIVE WITH NEUROPATHY ANYMORE!

>Dr. John Coppola, DC, ACN
>Dr. Valerie Monteiro Coppola, DC, CCST, ACN

>www.neuropathydoctorsa.com

INTRODUCTION

Oh! My Aching Feet!

As you sit in your living room, dreading the thought of having to get up to walk to the bathroom, your daughter or granddaughter comes waltzing in wearing her five-inch, high-heeled stiletto shoes, proclaiming, "OMG! My feet are killing me. I swear, *they're about to fall off!*" She yanks off her shoes, rubs her feet, wiggles her toes, and then jumps up and runs to the kitchen to grab something to eat. That's the extent of her foot pain. Oh, those were the days, weren't they? Remember when you could stand on your feet for hours without any pain? Do you remember when you could bounce out of your chair without a second thought? Now, you live in a world of constant pain and *strange* symptoms. You notice this weird tingling or numbness in your feet or hands. You feel stinging or electrical shocks in your legs. The soles of your feet feel like they are *on fire,* or your feet might be so sensitive that you can't even tolerate the weight of your bed sheet on them at night.

Throughout all of this, the unyielding pain limits your activities and disrupts your sleep. You've tried over-the-counter medication and sleep aids, which didn't work. Now, completely bewildered and at a loss for options, you visit your doctor, who diagnoses you with peripheral neuropathy and prescribes a medication like gabapentin (Neurontin). After taking it for a while, you realize that the medication hasn't helped, and the side effects you've encountered from the meds are worse than the original neuropathy symptoms.

You are not alone, and you are not crazy! It is estimated that **twenty-two million Americans are affected each year by peripheral neuropathy.** As a matter of fact, statistics show that **one out of every five people will be afflicted** by this disorder. What makes peripheral neuropathy seem like an elusive phantom? It's the fact that it has a wide variety of symptoms associated with it. For instance, your uncle might have peripheral neuropathy and complain that his feet feel like they are on fire, or your neighbor might complain that her neuropathy feels like she's walking on broken glass. You might also hear from others that they have only experienced mild numbness and tingling in their hands. The reason for this is that neuropathy can be caused by a vast number of different conditions. Diseases like diabetes cause some cases of neuropathy; other cases are caused by the use of prescription medications, like cholesterol meds or statin drugs. Still other cases of neuropathy might result from surgery. These are just a few of the things that can cause neuropathy.

Peripheral neuropathy can range from a mild annoyance to a life-threatening condition. I have a patient whose neuropathy in his arms is so severe that it has caused partial paralysis. Some of my patients are at risk for falls and fractures because of leg weakness and imbalance. What many folks don't realize is that peripheral neuropathy is not just limited to your arms and hands or legs and feet. It can also affect your vital organs,

INTRODUCTION

such as your heart, which can lead to arrhythmias, or your bladder, which can result in incontinence.

The following sections in this book will educate you about what neuropathy is as well as what you can do to be whole again. Unfortunately, many of you will read this book but neglect to take any action to change your condition. You will justify your complacency by telling yourself that this is too good to be true. Your condition can't possibly be reversed. These excuses will stand in your way of taking the necessary responsibility to get started. Don't let yourself be one of those people who suffer with this affliction because you are afraid to try something different. You are not alone in this quest. ***There is hope for your recovery.*** Let's get educated about what you can do for yourself or your loved one now!

PATIENT TESTIMONIALS

Francisco

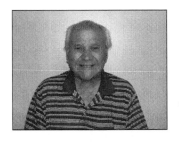

'I had been suffering from severe neuropathy, which limited my ability to sit, stand, and walk. What else is there to do besides sit, stand, and walk? To make matters worse, I couldn't get any sleep because the pain was so bad. I was prescribed gabapentin, which provided no relief and made me feel horrible.

When I started treatment at the San Antonio Neuropathy Center, I had my doubts that it would work. Within three treatments, the pain started to diminish. It was like a miracle for me. Today, I can enjoy the small pleasures of life, such as sitting, taking a walk, and enjoying a good night of sleep completely pain free. I would highly recommend the treatment to anyone who's suffering from neuropathy.

Maria

I am diabetic and I have suffered with neuropathy for ten years. The pain started off so mild and intermittent that I kept

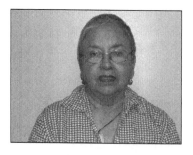 thinking it would go away on its own. Eventually, the pain and burning became so severe that I had to soak my feet in an ice-water bath just to get some relief.

Initially, I sought help from a podiatrist, since it was my feet that were being affected. He prescribed gabapentin and a lidocaine ointment. The medication provided very little relief, and it made me feel foggy. I know this sounds crazy, but the pain was so severe at times that I wanted my doctor to amputate some of my toes. The quality of my life was worse than poor, to say the least. There was never a time when I wasn't hobbling around in pain.

I heard about Dr. Coppola's neuropathy program and decided to give it a try. I had hit rock bottom and I had nothing to lose. After just two visits, I couldn't believe how dramatically my pain had been reduced. It was amazing. I didn't think anything could work that quickly.

After completing the program, I feel wonderful. The quality of my life has improved tremendously. I have started exercising, and I am now walking daily. To people who ask me am I happy with my decision to undergo Dr. Coppola's neuropathy program, I have only three words to say: Yes! Yes! Yes!

Rita

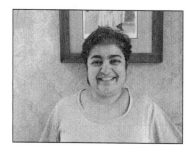 I began to slowly develop neuropathy over a period of four years. It started out as a feeling of numbness and tingling that would come and go. Eventually, the burning

became so intense that it would cause me to limp. As a chef, I needed to be on my feet for up to ten hours a day. By the end of the day, my pain was excruciating.

When my neuropathy began to interfere with my ability to work, I decided to see Dr. Coppola and Dr. Monteiro. They came highly recommended to me, but I still had doubts. I had previously seen several doctors, and no one was able to help me. After several treatments, my pain was substantially reduced. As the treatment progressed, the burning, numbness, and tingling subsided. Today, I'm able to work a full ten hours without any pain. I am so grateful for Dr. Coppola & Dr. Monteiro. I feel like I have my feet back!

Homer

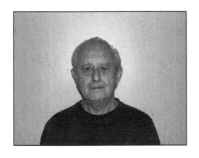

Several years ago, I started developing severe pain in my right calf and foot, and it later spread to my left foot. The pain in my toes was constant and so sharp that I could hardly stand it. The pain limited my ability to stand or walk for any length of time. I tried different medications and physical therapy, which didn't work. Finally, out of desperation, I went to see a neurosurgeon, who operated on my spine. Much to my dismay, the surgery provided no relief.

After reading some educational information provided by the San Antonio Neuropathy Center, I decided to go see them. The doctor took his time to really listen to my concerns. I began the neuropathy program, and after four treatments I began to feel significant improvement. Since the end of my treatment plan, my pain is completely gone. I still have some mild residual numbness, but that is gradually fading. I am thrilled with my results!

Basilia

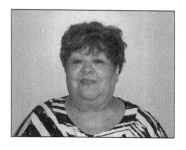

I had been suffering from neuropathy for two years. My feet were completely numb, and I would also experience pins and needles, burning, and sharp, shooting pain. I went to an endocrinologist who diagnosed me with borderline diabetes. I later saw a neurologist who attributed the nerve damage to my diabetes.

I tried different medications and physical therapy, which did not work. In fact, the medications made me feel worse. I couldn't stand, sit, or walk for more than thirty minutes without the onset of severe pain. It was really affecting the quality of my life.

I decided to begin the neuropathy treatment with Dr. Coppola, and within three treatments the pain was reduced, and I could stand and walk for longer periods. After completing the treatment, the pain is gone, and I can actually feel my feet again! I feel like my feet are coming to life again.

Sonja

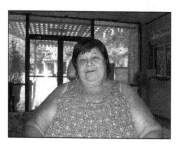

I had been suffering from neuropathy for seven years. I experienced numbness, tingling, and pain in my feet. Sometimes, it felt like I had a thousand needles piercing my feet. The numbness was so severe that I couldn't feel anything under my feet—not even the floor. As a result, my balance was extremely bad, forcing me to be bound to a wheelchair. I couldn't exercise, walk, or do anything to enjoy my life. I had tried different kinds of pain pills to control my pain, but nothing helped. I started water therapy, but I saw no results from that either. I felt hopeless, and I began to feel extremely depressed.

When I first learned about the program at the San Antonio Neuropathy Center, it sounded too good to be true. I had already tried so many other things that I didn't really believe that this program would work, but reluctantly, I gave it a try. After all, I had run out of options. Within just the first few treatments, I began to feel some sensation in my feet. It had literally been years since I felt *anything* on my feet. I was thrilled, as well, that the pain was dramatically reduced.

I am pleased to say that now I am walking around my house without the use of my motorized wheelchair. I have also begun to exercise again. I hadn't been able to do that for years.

My pain is completely gone! I am ecstatic and thrilled with my results. I recommend the doctors at San Antonio Neuropathy Center to everyone. They are excellent. I love the fact that the whole staff is very knowledgeable, professional, and caring.

Melvin

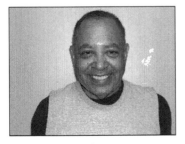

After having back surgery in 2005, I suffered from unrelenting neuropathy in my feet. The neuropathy started out gradually but then became progressively worse with time. It finally reached the point of being debilitating.

I suffered from severe pain and numbness in my feet whenever I would stand, walk, or even drive. At night, I would get horribly intense cramps in my lower legs and toes. It was so bad that it prevented me from getting a good night's sleep. I couldn't do laundry, mop the floor, or iron my clothes without difficulty and pain. My home was in disarray.

I went back to the doctor who had performed my original back surgery, and his solution was to perform a second back surgery. You've got to be kidding me, right? Needless to say, that wasn't even an option, after what I had gone through with my first back surgery.

Fortunately, I heard about some revolutionary new treatment at the San Antonio Neuropathy Center. I was a bit skeptical and nervous, but I was interested to learn more. I met with Dr. Coppola, who took the time to educate me about my condition. He didn't just throw the usual meds at me or tell me that I just needed to learn to live with my condition. I wasn't just another number with him. You could tell that he really cared and wanted me to understand what was going on with my nerves. I was excited to get started with the program.

After a few treatments, I felt encouraged as the pain started to subside, and my mobility improved. I was able to do simple chores, drive without pain, and walk for longer periods without limitations again. My quality of life really began to improve.

I now feel like I have my life back! I am absolutely thrilled that I completed Dr. Coppola's program, and I highly recommend it to anyone who's tired of succumbing to the debilitating effects of pain. I would rate the professionalism of the doctors and support staff at the highest degree. They put me at ease, and they were always eager to help. It was the first time in a long time that I felt like a doctor was interested in me—not just my wallet. I am truly grateful for Dr. Coppola.

Maurice

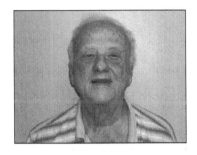

I have suffered from neuropathy for a long time. It affected both my hands and my feet. I experienced severe numbness and tingling in my toes and hands. It was so extreme that I had very little use of my hands. The pain would get so bad that it prevented me from sleeping, and as a result I suffered from sleep deprivation.

One of the few enjoyments in life that I had was volunteering for my church, where I helped out with odd jobs. I no longer was able to do much because I would lose my balance while standing or walking, and I would drop things due to the numbness in my hands and feet.

The only treatment that my doctor offered me was physical therapy, which was of very little help. So, I began searching for an alternative therapy to medication and physical therapy. Fortunately, I discovered the San Antonio Neuropathy Center. They offered me hope with their treatment plan. Within a few short weeks, the pain, numbness, and tingling were gone. It was amazing.

Since finishing my care, I have regained my balance, and I don't suffer from the risk of falling anymore. I have recovered the strength in my hands, and I can actually hold onto items. I have started volunteering my time at my church again, and I actually feel productive.

I am sleeping well again, and my energy levels are much better. Everyone at San Antonio Neuropathy Center has been excellent, and I am so appreciative that they have helped me live a normal life again. Thank you.

CATHY

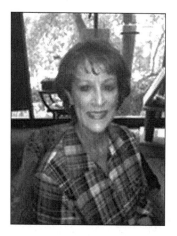

I first began my treatment with Dr. Coppola for my neuropathy. Although I was physically capable of walking, my neuropathy pain would get so bad that I would be forced to use a wheelchair. I had extreme numbness in my feet, ankles, and knees. I constantly felt like I had a tight band wrapped around the top of my knee by my thigh muscle. Between my pain and all of my other symptoms, this played a huge role in my inability to walk. I would also experience stabbing, sharp pains and severe spasms in my thighs. The pain was so crippling that it prevented me from driving, so I had to be chauffeured by my husband, family members, or friends to get anywhere, including my doctors' appointments.

After my first visit with Dr. Coppola, he told me that he would accept my case, but it would be difficult because my neuropathy was so advanced that it had begun to affect my organ systems like my heart, stomach, intestines, and bladder. He told me that I would also need to meet with Dr. Monteiro to co-manage my case. He explained to me that Dr. Monteiro's specialty was functional medicine. This meant that she would be supporting the function of my organ systems with nutrition, enabling them to heal, while Dr. C. worked on repairing my nerve function. I wasn't certain that it was even possible for me to recover, but I was desperate, and I wasn't ready to give up. I hated living this way. It seemed like not a single system was operating correctly in my body. It almost felt as if my body was just quitting on me.

After meeting with Dr. Monteiro, I felt a sense of hope for the first time on that dark path that I had been traveling. She understood my condition, but more important, she educated me about my own condition, and told me what it would take to turn it around. She assessed the medication that I was on and educated me about how it was contributing to my neuropathy, as well as my other organ dysfunctions. I was taking Nadolol for high blood pressure, which she told me was a beta blocker. She enlightened me about the dangers of beta blockers and their side effects, and then directed me to the *Drugs.com* website to learn more. My own doctor had *never* taken the time to do this for me.

Dr. Monteiro changed my diet and provided me with really delicious recipes. She put me on a juicing regimen and specific supplements to help support my organ functions. She also placed me on a detoxification program. The detox program was four weeks long and very restrictive. I honestly didn't know if I could do it. Fortunately, with all of her help and support, and the support of the staff, it was actually easier than I thought it would be.

After the first week of the detox, I noticed that my energy levels were great! I couldn't believe it. For the longest time, I was very self-conscious about red blotches that I had all over my face and neck; but for the first time in years they had completely disappeared. The stabbing pain and spasms in my upper thighs had completely stopped. By week three of the detox program, I had a follow-up appointment with my medical doctor, who ran lab tests on me. He was extremely impressed with the results of my lab work. It was the best it had ever been. I told him I wanted to stop taking nadolol. He didn't want to take me off this horrible drug. Fortunately, I brought in the page of side effects that I had printed up from Drugs.com and showed it to him. You could clearly see that the side effects and some of my symptoms overlapped. I held my ground firmly, and reluctantly he took me off of the drug.

I have now finished my detox program, and I could not be more pleased with the results. I no longer experience crippling pain. The tightness above my knees is completely gone. The numbness in my feet and ankles has improved, and I have increased sensations in them. I'm out of my wheelchair and using a cane. I've even begun to drive short distances.

I still have a way to go to be completely recovered, but I'm off to an amazing start. I now believe that recovery is very possible, and I have both Dr. Coppola and Dr. Monteiro to thank for that. They've given me back hope, belief, and the excitement to live every day!

Mary Lou

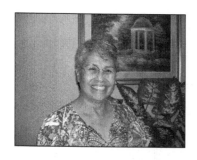

My occupation in housekeeping requires me to be very active on my feet all day. I began experiencing pain on the bottoms of my feet and in my hands. The pain was always very intense, but the type of pain would often change. Sometimes my pain would be sharp and shooting. At other times, I would experience swelling in my legs and feet with strong cramping and dull aches. There were also occasions when my feet would feel like they were on fire. The intensity would get so bad that it would limit my activity level significantly. Prior to this pain, I could work through the morning until lunch without slowing down. Because I've been suffering from this pain, I would have to take two to three breaks during my morning shift, which would slow me down considerably. The pain also sapped all of my energy.

Since I've had a history of cardiac issues, I vowed to walk thirty-five to forty-five minutes a day, thinking that this might improve my energy and health. This only worsened the pain in my feet, and I also began to develop pain in my back and hips. It would get so bad, I couldn't even walk.

I went to my medical doctor for these conditions. All they did was prescribe Celebrex and recommend that I take Advil. I didn't want to become dependent on these meds, so I only took them when it was absolutely necessary. Seven months later, my condition had continued to worsen. Around this time, I read about Dr. John Coppola and his nonsurgical treatments for neuropathy and back conditions, so I scheduled an appointment with him.

After doing a thorough work-up on me, Dr. Coppola diagnosed me with neuropathy and prescribed a treatment plan consisting of nonsurgical spinal decompression for my back pain and hip and neurocare for my neuropathy pain. Dr. Coppola placed me on several supplements to help my nerves heal. He also educated me and eased me into making healthier eating choices.

I couldn't believe how comfortable and relaxing my treatments were. At first, I noticed gradual results, but with time they became increasingly obvious. After my tenth treatment, the pain in my feet and back had diminished substantially, allowing me to take walks again. I was now able to walk for twenty to twenty-five minutes. This was remarkable, because I hadn't been able to walk in three months. I never thought this would be possible, and I'm so grateful for Dr. C. and his caring staff!

"*The first step in natural healing is responsibility. Natural healing is about taking control of your life and being responsible for everything that goes in and out of your body, mind, and spirit.*"

—Dr. Richard Schulze

"*Every human being is the author of his own health or disease.*"

—Buddha

1

THE GREAT NEUROPATHY HOAX

*"He who has health has hope;
and he who has hope, has everything."*

Thomas Carlisle
(1795–1881)

I'm sorry. You have peripheral neuropathy. There is no cure or solution for it. We don't know what causes it, but I can prescribe some medication to help you with your symptoms. It will get worse with time, and this is something that you need to accept. You are going to have to learn to live with this condition...

Does this sound familiar to you? It is what doctors commonly tell most neuropathy sufferers, and it is the biggest pile of *bull*.

A neuropathy diagnosis is mysterious and elusive. The onset of neuropathy is insidious, occurring very slowly with time and then rapidly advancing in later stages. Most medical doctors will tell you that the cause is idiopathic, which means that its origin is unknown. In truth, this means that the doctor simply has not discovered the origin. This is typically because the doctor does not read or understand the scientific literature, or they are too busy to research the cause. Instead, we find teams of medical professionals being influenced by propaganda, which includes manipulated research produced by the pharmaceutical companies.

The reality is that there are a number of causes leading to peripheral neuropathy that we *do* know about. The problem is that the causes of neuropathy are rarely simple or easily identifiable. Neuropathy is very seldom caused by just one factor. There are usually two, three, or more factors that have contributed to the onset of your condition. Herein lays the challenge. It can, in fact, be time-consuming to investigate and uncover your specific causes.

For this reason it is imperative that you become a *Sherlock Holmes* for your condition. You must be proactive and do some basic research for yourself. You cannot solely rely on your doctor. I understand that this thought terrifies you, but your health and your life depend upon it. Since you don't have the luxury of grabbing a seat in the bleachers or merely sitting along the sidelines, we are here to help guide you. We will provide you with the most current and objective research findings. I applaud you for beginning to take responsibility, by picking up this book. The next step is to educate yourself enough so that you only need to utilize your doctor for guidance and direction—as a roadmap, 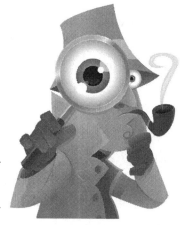 if you will. If you fail to educate yourself about your condition, you will not know what questions to ask. Even when given a roadmap, you chart a course with the knowledge that it is still up to you to keep your eyes wide open while traveling—especially if this is a new and uncharted road for you. You must be on the lookout for roadblocks, detours, or potholes along the way. The same holds true for your journey with your health.

Unfortunately, you cannot rely upon your medical doctor to do this for you. In today's world of managed health care, doctors are akin to hamsters on a wheel, spinning incessantly to meet the overhead of their clinic. This means they must treat a higher volume of patients, leaving little time for each patient. This is one of the largest reasons that there is a sky rocketing number of mistakes (some tragic) made by doctors and hospitals. It is unwise to turn complete control of your health over to your doctor. Following your doctor's instructions or recommendations blindly, without taking the time to learn about your condition, will render you unable to ask appropriate questions. After all, do you blindly turn complete control of your hard-earned money—your life's savings—over to someone you barely know simply because they have impressive-looking credentials?–of course not. The reality is that we safeguard our money more than we do our health.

This doesn't mean that your doctor doesn't care about you or your condition; it simply means that they are struggling to keep their heads above water. This is mainly why, when you walk into your doctor's office, you find it packed—possibly standing room only. How common is it for you to have to wait for an hour before the doctor can see you? This alone makes it difficult—and sometimes impossible—for doctors to stay up-to-date on the latest unbiased research. Remember when you were a student? It was much easier for you when you had a course in which the teacher spoon-fed you the answers, as opposed to expecting you to go out and search for them yourself. Well, pharmaceutical companies are all too eager to spoon-feed your doctor the answers—they throw the doctors a life preserver, and many are all too willing to latch on. In the United States, there are an estimated eighty thousand drug company representatives who visit doctors every day. These pharmaceutical reps are backed by more than $19 billion of combined promotional yearly budgets that they lavish on the doctors. All of this is designed to influence your doctor so that he or she will favor the particular drugs that the rep is touting.

> **Pharmaceutical Reps**
>
> Most representatives of the pharmaceutical companies have degrees in marketing, sociology, or psychology (social sciences).

Most physicians are well-intentioned individuals who wholeheartedly believe that they are doing the best they can for their patients. They are oblivious to the fact that they are merely pawns in a pharmaceutical system that spends tens of billions of dollars *every year* deceiving them into believing that drugs are the best solution. The sad truth is that although your doctor cares very much about you, the pharmaceutical rep doesn't know you or give a damn about you. The rep's main concern is filling their quota for the month and making their bonus. It is not uncommon for their bonus to be larger than their actual salary. By the way, the pharmaceutical representative is not a medical professional. They are people who have undergraduate Bachelor of Science degrees in marketing or social science. Social science does not include standard science classes like biology, chemistry, or physics (courses required for students seeking to enter a medical profession). On the contrary, the social sciences incorporate psychology, sociology, political science, and education, to name a few. It is concerning that the pharmaceutical rep, who is educating your doctor on this wonder drug they are pushing, has a degree in marketing, rather than chemistry. This means that pharmaceutical reps are competent at selling their products. This is a bonus for the pharmaceutical company, rather than for the patient or the doctor. Needless to say, this is troubling. As a result, your doctor is being blindly led down a self-serving road to be sold a bill of goods, which may or may not help you. Worse yet, it might harm you. Do you think that I am overreacting? Let's visit a list of drugs that were approved by the FDA over the past ten years only to be withdrawn later from the market because these drugs caused serious illnesses—such as strokes and heart attacks—and even death.

This table is available at www.worstpills.org. This is a very informative website that is aimed at educating consumers about drugs with the safest track records and those with the worst track records. I often use this website to educate my patients about the medications that they might be taking.

Twenty Drugs Approved After 1992 and Later Withdrawn From the Market for Safety Reasons (Starting With the Most Recent Withdrawals)

No	Generic Name (BRAND NAME)	Date of US approval	Date of US withdrawal	Time on the Market
20	sibutramine (MERIDIA)	11/22/1997	10/8/2010	12.9 years
19	efalizumab (RAPTIVA)	10/28/2003	4/8/2009	5.5 years
18	trasylol (APROTININ)	12/29/1993	11/5/2007	3.9 years
17	tegaserod (ZELNORM)	7/24/2002	3/30/2007	4.7 years

No	Generic Name (BRAND NAME)	Date of US approval	Date of US withdrawal	Time on the Market
16	gatifloxacin (TEQUIN)	12/17/1999	5/1/2006	6.4 years
15	technetium (99m TC) fanolesomab (NEUTROSPEC)	7/2/2004	12/19/2005	1.5 years
14	hydromorphone (PALLADONE)	9/24/2004	7/13/2005	0.8 years
13	valdecoxib (BEXTRA)	11/16/2001	4/7/2005	3.4 years
12	natalizumab (TYSABRI)	11/23/2004	2/28/2005	0.3 years
11	rofecoxib (VIOXX)	5/20/1999	9/29/2004	5.4 years
10	levomethadyl (ORLAAM)	7/9/1993	9/2/2003	10.2 years
9	cerivastatin (BAYCOL)	6/26/1997	8/8/2001	7.3 years
8	rapacuronium (RAPLON)	8/18/1999	3/30/2001	1.6 years
7	alosetron (LOTRONEX)	2/9/2000	11/28/2000	0.8 years
6	cisapride (PROPULSID)	7/29/1993	3/24/2000	9.7 years
5	troglitazone (REZULIN)	1/29/1997	3/21/2000	3.1 years
4	grepafloxacin (RAXAR)	11/6/1997	8/11/1999	1.8 years
3	bromfenac (DURACT)	7/15/1997	6/22/1998	0.9 years
2	mibefradil (POSICOR)	6/20/1997	6/8/1998	1.0 years
1	dexfenfluramine (REDUX)	6/1/1996	9/15/1997	1.3 years

Now, I don't want you to think that I have anything against pharmaceutical reps. As a matter of fact, I know a few of them personally, and the ones I know are really outstanding people. However, although these people might be highly qualified to market medications, they are not qualified to educate any doctor on the mechanisms and roles of these drugs. Think about it. How comfortable would you feel if you went to a doctor whose degree was in marketing, rather than medical science? Would you let them treat you?

Would you even be interested in anything that this doctor had to say? Why don't these pharmaceutical reps come from the medical field? I don't know about you, but this is pretty mind-boggling to me.

Reviewing medical research is labor intensive and can be downright confusing. If you are going to spend time sifting through research, you must be able to discern which is biased (i.e., paid for by a company that has an agenda and directly benefits from the outcome) and which is completely untainted. It is no easy task. As you begin to take control of your health and sift through the vast array of information on the Internet, your head will begin to spin.

One website might say, "Neuropathy is permanent." Another site might say that it is not permanent. You will come across a site that states, "Take this drug to alleviate your neuropathy pain," yet a second site might point out all of the adverse side effects of taking this drug. Don't go running for the hills in confusion just yet. I am here to help shed some light on this subject for you.

Our role along your journey is to give you clarity about your peripheral neuropathy. It is our desire to provide you with information about your condition that you will not receive from your doctor—not even your neurologist. This will aid you in charting your course. It is our goal to make you aware of what to look for in treatment and diagnosis, and about other factors that might actually be worsening your neuropathy. We want to empower you so that you can make the most informed decisions on your own. To do this, let's take a look at some common myths you might have been told about neuropathy.

DEBUNKING THE BULL YOU'VE BEEN SOLD!

Myth #1: Medication will cure my neuropathy.

- **False.** The most common treatment for neuropathy is the...take-some-pills-and-wait-and-see method.

- Some of the more common drugs given include Hydrocodone, gabapentin (Neurontin), pregabalin (Lyrica), duloxetine (Cymbalta), and Tramodol—all of which have serious side effects. While this may be necessary for the temporary relief of severe symptoms, the truth is that **medications do absolutely nothing to reverse nerve damage.** In fact, some medications, such as gabapentin, actually accelerate the nerve damage.

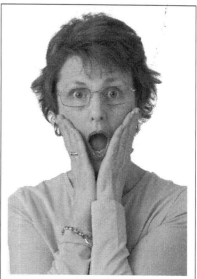

It may shock you to find out you have been sold "horse manure." Let's debunk these common myths.

Myth #2: Neuropathy only affects people with diabetes.

- **False.** Actually, diabetic patients account for less than 20 percent of all neuropathy cases. There are far more neuropathy sufferers that are not diabetes related, according to a 2009 study. A study published by the Neuropathy Association revealed the following findings:

"Neuropathy is often misrepresented as only being diabetes-related. However, this survey demonstrates that for every diabetic neuropathy patient, there are at least six more patients suffering with other various forms of neuropathies."

Dr. Thomas H. Brannagan, III
(medical advisor for the Neuropathy Association)

While neuropathy is common in diabetic patients, there are many other causes of neuropathy. Some common causes include: chemotherapy, B-vitamin deficiency, nerve damage or entrapment, and side effects associated with commonly prescribed medications. If you feel pain, even if you're not diabetic, your neuropathy may be due to one or more of the causes listed above.

Myth #3: My doctor told me, "Nerves don't regenerate. once damaged…that's it!"

- **False.** Your doctor is not up-to-date on the current research. There are extensive studies revealing the contrary. The research covers a wide array of therapies, including neurotropic nutrients, low-level laser therapy, exercise, and nutrition. To learn more details, you will need to read further on in this book, as this is an extensive topic.

Myth #4: I only have numbness and tingling, so it's no big deal.

- **False.** Many neuropathy patients who suffer from mild numbness or tingling think that their symptoms are no big deal. They don't understand that what they are feeling is only the tip of the iceberg. They think because they can continue to function—*business as usual*—the numbness and tingling will fade away all by itself without any treatment.

But a study in the *British Medical Journal* proved this myth false, showing that **75 percent of sufferers who do nothing about the numbness and tingling will have either pain or disability twelve months later**. Let's face it, if your neuropathy symptoms haven't gone away by now, it's not likely they will disappear on their own. And it has been shown in studies that if ignored, symptoms can intensify, causing loss of sensation, unremitting pain, and even disability.

Myth #5: Neuropathy is a natural result of aging.

- **False.** You can grow old gracefully without ever experiencing these levels of nerve damage. Neuropathy, once known only in the senior sector, is now affecting people as young as thirty years old. This disorder can be caused by injuries, chronic illnesses, and complications caused by medications, among other things. By taking the right steps early on, you can avoid suffering from many neuropathic symptoms as you get older.

Myth #6: I have to accept my neuropathy and learn to live with it.

- **False:** Neuropathy doesn't have to be a life sentence. A combination of proper stimulation of your nerves at home and in the clinic, detox, glucose control, and appropriate nutrients plays a pivotal role in nerve repair and regeneration. Whatever you do, don't go untreated!

Myth #7: All neuropathy feels the same.

- **False:** Neuropathy symptoms can vary dramatically, depending on the cause and the stage of neuropathy. We know that there are many causes of neuropathy (see Myth #2). Early-stage neuropathy symptoms are typically mild numbness and tingling, whereas late-stage neuropathy can show up as creepy-crawly sensations, sharp pains, a loss of balance, and even significant muscle weakness. An unhappy nerve can't communicate as well to the brain, and the brain misinterprets the signals as all kinds of different symptoms.

Myth #8: My neuropathy is well-controlled by medications, so I'm doing just fine.

- **False:** Medications merely mask symptoms, while the underlying condition continues to get worse. Medicating the symptoms is like taking the battery out of your smoke alarm to stop the noise.

Your pain might be gone, but the meds might be hiding a gradual loss of nerve function, and you could be losing your ability to maintain good balance. Then one day, without warning, you might fall and break your arm—or worse, a hip. Remember, if your neuropathy is not getting better, it's probably getting worse.

Myth #9: Neuropathy only affects the hands and feet.

- **False:** Although neuropathy often begins in the hands and feet, it will eventually slowly creep up the calves and forearms. Oftentimes, this can present itself as severe cramps, heaviness, or weakness in the legs, a creepy-crawly sensation, and a dry discoloration of the skin. In some cases, neuropathy can even cause dangerous complications in organ function.

Myth #10: The best thing to do for my neuropathy is to wait and see what happens.

- **False:** This is by far the worst thing you can do. The consensus of the professional healthcare community, including top neurologists, oncologists and surgeons, all agree that peripheral neuropathy rarely, if ever, improves on its own. More often than not, the condition continues to worsen and can become debilitating. By detecting and treating neuropathy early on, you are more likely to have a much better prognosis. That's not to say that more advanced neuropathy cannot be resolved. However, people with more advanced neuropathy tend to need more care, and the results tend to be slower.

Warning

Never discontinue the use of a prescribed medication without being instructed to do so by your physician.

Prescription medications cannot be stopped abruptly.

2

LIES YOUR DRUG COMPANY DOESN'T WANT YOU TO KNOW ABOUT

"The best doctor gives the least medicines."

Benjamin Franklin
(1706-1790)

The standard treatment for peripheral neuropathy is prescription medications. Since your doctor has already informed you that there is no cure for neuropathy, their only course of action is to attempt to manage your pain and symptoms. There are several commonly prescribed drugs that are being used to treat neuropathy:

- Neurontin/gabapentin
- Cymbalta/duloxetine
- Lyrica/pregabalin
- Epitol/carbamazepine

Ironically, not one of these drugs was approved by the Food and Drug Administration (FDA) for the treatment of neuropathy or nerve conditions. When a doctor writes a prescription to treat your neuropathy, it's not unreasonable for you to assume that the drug that he or she is prescribing has been approved and regulated by the FDA to treat the condition that you have, neuropathy. That would be a reasonable assumption, but as in these cases, it is not always true. These drugs are often being used for the treatment of neuropathy, which is called off-label use.

Let's explore what off-labeling means. To do this, it is important for you to understand how a drug is labeled and what this means for you. In the US, new drugs are tested in clinical trials, which are also known as research studies, before they are approved for use by the general public. The clinical trials are performed to prove that the drug does the following:

- Works to treat a specific medical condition.
- Works the way it is intended to work.
- Is safe when used as directed.

When the FDA is satisfied that a drug has been through extensive trials and research proving its efficacy and safety for public use, it will work with the maker of the drug to create a drug label. The initial drug label includes very specific information about which medical conditions the drug was approved for and the approved doses of the medication. Once the FDA approves this report, the drug is then made available to all health professionals, who prescribe or sell the drug.

When a drug is used in any way that is different from what is described in the FDA-approved drug label, it is said to be an off-label use. Off-labeling may mean that the drug is being:

- used for a different medical condition than what was originally approved by the FDA
- administered via different route (oral, IV, topical, etc.)
- administered in a different dose than the label indicates

The use of off-label drugs by medical doctors is not regulated, but it is legal in the United States. According to an article published in the prestigious *New England Journal of Medicine* in 2008, off-labeling is becoming a problematic and dangerous practice. They state, "Although off-label prescribing—the prescription of a medication in a manner different from that approved by the FDA—is legal and common, it is often done in the absence of adequate supporting data. Off-label uses have not been formally evaluated, and evidence provided for one clinical situation may not apply to others.

"A 2003 report showed that off-label use accounted for approximately 21% of all prescriptions. The highest rates of off-label use were for anticonvulsants (many of which are used to treat neuropathic pain) antipsychotics, and antibiotics. ***Most off-label drug uses were shown to have little or no scientific support.*** Antipsychotics and antidepressants were particularly likely to be used off-label without strong evidence."

> 73 percent of off-label drug uses were shown to have little or NO scientific support.

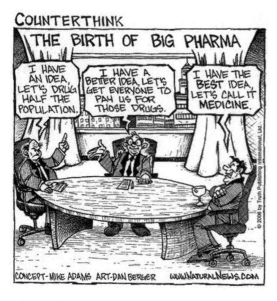

So, let's examine some of the commonly prescribed off-label drugs for neuropathy. Cymbalta is an antidepressant drug that is prescribed off-label for neuropathy. I guess one approach to neuropathy is to try to make your nerves more cheerful. When I questioned a few of my patients who were currently taking Cymbalta, they had no idea that it was an antidepressant. They stated, "My doctor said I had to take this for my neuropathy pain." When I informed them that this medication was an antidepressant, one gentleman stated, "So, will it make my nerves happier, then?" He's a humorous man in spite of his neuropathy, and we both chuckled over that one. When I asked my patients who were seeking help for their neuropathy if the Cymbalta helped their pain, they resoundingly answered no. This didn't surprise me, though; if it had helped them, they likely wouldn't have been in my office. So my next question was: "Then why are you still taking the Cymbalta?" Their response was one that I often hear: "My doctor didn't want to take me off it." The patient left it at that and called it a day. As incredible as this may seem, it is quite commonplace, unfortunately. The one thing that I can tell you is that this is not typically because the doctor is uncaring. The opposite is usually true—your doctor is very caring and wants to see you get better. This scenario is usually because of the hamster-on-the-wheel syndrome that I mentioned earlier. Your doctor is spread so thin that he or she overlooked the fact that Cymbalta had not provided you any pain relief, which should have been the cue to take you off the medication. Cymbalta is prescribed for people suffering from clinically diagnosed major depressive disorder (MDD) and generalized anxiety disorder (GAD). It should not be used to help you deal with the normal, daily stresses of life. Whether you are using Cymbalta for depression or anxiety, or off-label to manage pain, it is important to know the possible side effects of this medication. Cymbalta has been shown to cause a worsening of depression in some people. It can also increase a risk for developing suicidal thoughts or actions in those already suffering from depression or other mental disorders. Other reported side effects include liver damage, jaundice, vomiting, flu-like symptoms, itching, and dark-colored urine.

The next group of medications prescribed for neuropathy is actually anticonvulsant or antiepileptic medications. They are gabapentin (Neurontin), pregabalin (Lyrica), and carbamazepine (Epitol). The FDA has never approved any of these drugs for treating neuropathy. I won't address each of these drugs with you, but I will go over some facts and data for the most commonly prescribed off-label drug in treating neuropathy, Neurontin.

Gabapentin (Neurontin) — neuropathy medication

History: Japanese researchers discovered gabapentin over forty years ago. It was later sold to Parke-Davis (Warner-Lambert, Inc.), a subsidiary of Pfizer (the world's largest pharmaceutical company), who discovered its effectiveness in treating epilepsy and certain seizure disorders. Neurontin was first tested on humans in 1987. In 1993, the FDA approved it to be used *in conjunction* with other epilepsy drugs. It was not to be used as a stand-alone drug, because a significant side effect of the drug is that it can induce depression and suicidal thoughts in patients. This medication was then developed as a supplemental medication for other anticonvulsant drugs to help minimize and prevent seizures.

Neurontin was formulated after the neurotransmitter, GABA. GABA plays a role in regulating the excitability of neurons (or nerves) throughout the nervous system. GABA is also directly responsible for controlling muscle tone.

Here is the surprising part: no one knows how gabapentin (Neurontin) works. Teams of scientists can't explain how it offers pain relief or acts as an anticonvulsant. Despite the fact that Neurontin resembles GABA, it has no direct effect on the function or action of the nervous system. In addition, gabapentin does not affect dopamine or serotonin, other common neurotransmitters. The one effect that is known is that gabapentin has the ability to block the actions of calcium channels (channels that selectively allow calcium to pass into cells), which limits the availability of the calcium necessary for the proper function of the nerves. This creates a huge problem for the overall health of the nerve, which I will cover in greater detail in the section of calcium channel blocking drugs.

Neurontin (the trade name) and gabapentin (the generic name) are two of the more common names for this drug, but it also has several other brand names: FusePaq, Fanatrex, Gabarone, Gralise, and Nupentin. This product is available in tablet, capsule, and liquid form. Even though **the FDA has only approved this medication for use in seizures and post-herpetic** *neuralgia*, it has become the drug of choice in treating peripheral neuropathy. **It is still widely prescribed by doctors in spite of the mounting evidence showing that Neurontin has very little value as pain relief, and carries huge side effects.**

According to a study by Randall Stafford, MD, a medical professor at Stanford University in Palo Alto, California, a large percentage of all drug sales in the US are prescribed for unapproved uses without adequate evidence that the medicines work. He estimates that doctors write more than ten million prescriptions like this each year. As described earlier, medical doctors have the ability to prescribe drugs for off-label use when nothing else works for a condition. It is acknowledged, however, that off-label use of many drugs is problematic in the medical community. Although, the doctor is granted the ability to prescribe this medication when all else has failed, the law clearly stipulates that the pharmaceutical company cannot market it to the public or to doctors for any use other than what the FDA has approved. Sadly, this law is frequently disregarded by the pharmaceutical giants.

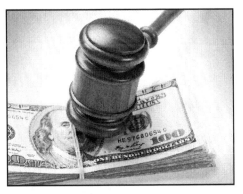

Pharmaceutical companies have openly showered doctors with cash to persuade them to use drugs off-label, according to many doctors' reports.

Peter Lurie is a physician and the deputy medical director of Public Citizen, a Washington-based public interest group. He has published articles in the acclaimed journals of the *Lancet* and the *Journal of the American Medical Association*

(*JAMA*). He states, "Doctors generally don't tell people that they're prescribing drugs pitched to them by pharmaceutical salespeople for unapproved treatments."

> **Research conducted by Pfizer – maker of Gabapentin**
>
> ▶ Study finds that placebo outperformed Neurontin/gabapentin in trials.

As a matter of fact, in 2004, one of the pharmaceutical giants, Warner-Lambert, a unit of Pfizer, pleaded guilty to two felony counts of illegal marketing of a drug for unapproved uses. Pfizer was found guilty of marketing gabapentin for uses that the **FDA never approved**, in particular, migraines, bipolar disorder and **neuropathic pain,** prosecutor Michael Loucks, head of the Health Care Fraud Unit reported.

Pfizer, the world's largest pharmaceutical company, pleaded guilty in 2004 and agreed to pay $430 million to resolve criminal and civil charges that it paid doctors to prescribe its epilepsy drug, Neurontin, to patients with ailments that the drug was not federally approved to treat. "They [Warner-Lambert] made their money, and they got off cheap," says Larry Sasich, a doctor of pharmacy at the consumer-oriented Public Citizen Health Research Group based in Washington, DC. Since the Warner-Lambert executives were not prosecuted, he says, the $430 million fine is an inexpensive "cost of doing business."

In March 2010, Pfizer was found guilty of further criminal actions upon revealing the fact that Pfizer's team of medical researchers had conducted studies on the efficacy of Neurontin (gabapentin) but then buried the findings. Why would they spend so much money on a research team and then not want to use the results? Their research studies showed that Neurontin was no more effective in treating neuropathy than the placebo.

In essence, taking a sugar pill was as effective in treating neuropathy as taking Neurontin. Just when you think it can't possibly get worse…it does. Furthermore, their research revealed that the use of gabapentin led to many harmful effects. The jury came back with a verdict against Pfizer for $47.4 million in damages, which was automatically tripled under the RICO Act's provisions, making the judgment a grand total of over $142 million.

Don't feel bad for this pharmaceutical company, though. As large as the penalties are for drug companies caught breaking the off-label law, the fines are tiny compared with the firms' annual revenues.

> In 1993, The FDA approved gabapentin (Neurontin) as a supplemental medication for treating epilepsy. This drug was never approved for the treatment of neuropathy.

Pfizer made $2.27 billion from sales of Neurontin in 2002. Ninety-four percent, or $2.12 billion, of this revenue directly resulted from off-label use, according to the prosecutors' 2004 Pfizer sentencing memo. To date, Pfizer continues to earn over $2 billion annually from sales of both Neurontin (brand name) and gabapentin (generic brand), as reported in Bloomberg's annual sales report. In fact, the total of $2.75 billion that Pfizer has paid in off-label penalties since 2004 is a little more than 1 percent of the company's revenue of $245 billion from 2004 to 2008.

"Marketing departments of many drug companies don't respect any boundaries of professionalism or the law," says Jerry Avorn, a professor at Harvard Medical School in Boston and author of *Powerful Medicines: The Benefits, Risks, and Costs of Prescription Drugs* (Random House, 2004).

You may wonder why medical doctors are still prescribing this drug. As a matter of fact, if you go back to your medical doctors and ask them about the efficacy of gabapentin, they will probably say, "It's a great drug for neuropathy." They will further tell you that a lot of research shows that the drug works. So, are your doctors lying to you? No. They are not lying. Dr. Lurie says, "Most physicians don't keep track of FDA-approved uses of drugs, and the great majority of doctors have no idea; they don't even understand the distinction between on- and off-labeling."

To complicate matters further, lots of research shows how great gabapentin is for treating neuropathy. When I began researching the contradicting conclusions of the opposing teams, it made my head spin.

> **NEURONTIN ~ GABAPENTIN**
>
> ~ Only approved by the FDA for use in treating seizures and post-herpetic neuralgia.
>
> ~ Research shows ineffective for neuropathy pain.

After all, why would one set of research show so clearly that this drug is ineffective while the other set shows that it is effective? Well, after conducting intensive research, I realized that the studies that demonstrated how amazing the results were for gabapentin were funded by—you guessed it—the pharmaceutical companies. They are very clever at disguising their funding in these research studies. They commonly open up nonprofit organizations under assumed names that go virtually undetected as the main source of funding.

Fortunately, I was able to find unbiased, untainted research studies on the efficacy of gabapentin. One study published in the *American Family Physician Journal* in 2006 found that gabapentin was ***completely ineffective for acute neuropathic pain*** and was only shown to have a mild to moderate effect—with extremely high dosages—in minimizing chronic neuropathic pain. The study used a wide variety of dosages starting at 900 mg per day up to 3,600 mg. For there to be even minimal relief in a minority of study participants, dosages of 1,800 mg per day had to be exceeded. Commonly, dosages of 2,400–3,600 mg were used (mind you, the maximum recommended dosage according to the labeling on the medication is 1,800 mg per day). This paper further pointed out that significant damage and side effects had been shown to occur at dosages exceeding 1,800 mg per day. These effects included dizziness, headaches, drowsiness, diarrhea, and confusion. Many patients who participated in a survey complained, "Neurontin made me feel like a zombie."

<u>Other</u> *common side effects of Neurontin are*

- Loss of balance and shaky movements
- Tremors or twitching muscles
- Numbness, pins and needles, or other altered sensations
- Fever
- Increased rate of infections
- Decrease in white blood cells
- Mood instability
- Confusion, memory loss, or amnesia
- Depression

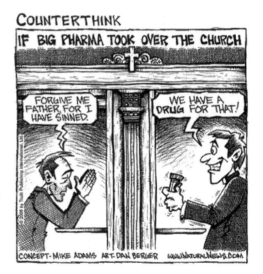

- Anxiety or nervousness
- Insomnia
- High blood pressure or elevated blood pressure
- Shortness of breath

Warning: If you are presently taking Neurontin, **do not stop taking it without consulting your physician**. A sudden reduction in dosage could cause seizures, so the dosage should be tapered gradually under your doctor's supervision.

I commonly find neuropathy sufferers taking seven or more medications for a variety of ailments, which may or may not include their neuropathy. One patient came to me who was taking twenty-one prescribed medications. I wish I could say that this patient was an isolated case, but unfortunately, I see this repeatedly.

I frequently encounter people who were placed on Neurontin for their neuropathy and developed symptoms of depression as a result. Then, their well-meaning doctor placed them on an antidepressant—and so the cascade began. You have neuropathy, and your doctor prescribes gabapentin for you. While on this medication, you experience depression, anxiety, and mood swings, so your doctor places you on an antidepressant such as Cymbalta. Then you develop high blood pressure, so your doctor places you on Norvasc. Now you can't sleep because of the pain and anxiety, so you are placed on Ambien. Before you know it—*BAM*—you are taking seven different prescriptions. "Sounds crazy!" you say. But it's not. It's quite common. You can clearly see that some of the side effects from this drug, gabapentin, are the same as the symptoms of your neuropathy, so in the end, it is possible that this drug has actually worsened your neuropathy.

DRUGS COMMONLY PRESCRIBED FOR OFF-LABEL USE

1. Anti-seizure drugs (Gabapentin) → Migraines, depression, nerve pain, hot flashes, fibromyalgia

2. Antidepressants (Cymbalta, Elavil) → Nerve pain, chronic pain, ADHD, bipolar disorder

3. Anxiety drugs → Normal life stresses, sleeping problems

4. Beta-Blockers → Migraines, heart rhythm disorders, anxiety

Note: *This excerpt is taken from Consumer Reports Best Buy Drugs. To view the entire article and list, go to:*

www.CRBestBuyDrugs.org

Here is what the article in Consumer Reports: Best Buy Drugs, Shopper's Guide to Prescription Drugs—Number 6: Off-Label Drug Use, had to say:

What Your Doctor Knows…Or Should!

"As is hopefully clear by now, doctors are major players in the off-label story. They wear white hats when they prescribe a drug off-label and it works well. They are also sometimes unwitting victims of drug-company marketing or false promotions of off-label uses—including informal office visits by drug company sales people.(1)

"But doctors can at times be the willful perpetrators of unsupported off-label use—when they should know better. (2)

"For example, the FDA has had rules, instituted in 1998, on precisely what sales representatives can say about the off-label use of a drug. They are permitted to share studies that have been published in reputable medical journals and that are going to be used to support a future application to the FDA for approval.(3)

"But many critics, state attorneys general, consumer organizations, and doctors themselves believe that the rules continue to be regularly violated, and that many doctors—during their busy days—don't bother to hold drug salespeople to the letter of the law.(4)

"In addition, studies over many years have shown that most doctors don't always know about the detailed labeling of a drug, and what its 'approved' use is. Rather, they rely on their colleagues and what is known as 'community standards of practice' in their prescribing habits."(5)

Here are a few questions to ask your doctor when you are being prescribed any medication. You need to decide for yourself whether or not you are willing to assume the risk of taking the medication. At the end of the day, you are the one who will suffer the consequences—not your doctor—regardless of how well intentioned they may be.

ASK YOUR DOCTOR THESE QUESTIONS ABOUT ANY PRESCRIBED MEDICATION

- Is this drug being used for an approved use or an off-label use? (You should be concerned if your doctor doesn't know. Be sure to ask your pharmacist the same question when filling the prescription.)

- If the doctor's response is that it's an off-label use, ask, "What has this drug been approved for?"

- If the prescription is off-label, ask your doctor whether scientific evidence supports this use, and ask which journal you could find this information in.

TAKE CONTROL

✓ Don't accept the following statement from either a doctor or pharmacist: "Don't worry; this drug is commonly prescribed off-label for this reason." Just because it is commonly used off-label doesn't mean that it's safe or even beneficial. Remember, the off-label use is an unapproved use. The FDA does not support off-label uses, and research often does not support it, either.

✓ Go online and research the drug. Drugs.com will give you good information. You can find labeling information on the FDA website **(http://www.accessdata.fda.gov/scripts/cder/drussatfda/).**

✓ You do not have to accept any medication that you don't feel comfortable taking. If you are uncomfortable, ask your doctor for a safer alternative. A doctor who truly cares about your health will also care about your concerns and will not try to bully you.

It is important to remember that there is *no* drug on the market currently that will reverse or heal your neuropathy. Any of the drugs used to treat neuropathy are prescribed only in an attempt to manage the symptoms. This is not to say that all medication is bad and useless. This clearly is not the case. Medications have their time and place. If you are among the minority of people whose pain has been alleviated by neuropathy medications, that's fantastic. As a doctor, a healer, I hate to see any person suffer. However, a vast majority of people have tried these drugs—or are still taking them—have not seen any results. All too often, people have suffered from the side effects of these drugs.

On the brighter side, as you continue reading, you will see that there are a number of ways that you can heal your damaged and inflamed nerves. Will this be easy? Nothing worthwhile ever is. However, I can tell you that it is very possible and doable. Will you recover from your neuropathy? Unfortunately, there are no guarantees that you will recover. However, more than 80 percent of people suffering from neuropathy have had tremendous results repairing and regenerating their nerves when they have followed the guidelines that I am laying out for you in this book. What was the key ingredient for them? Taking responsibility for their health and not waiting for someone else to do it for them.

You have already begun to take responsibility for your health by picking up this book. I commend you. I am not here to sell you anything. My main purpose is to educate you and return your hope to you. The pain and agony that you or a love one has been enduring does not have to be a way of life for the remainder of your life. It can be turned around, but this won't happen as the result of taking drugs. The road to recovery starts with you and your actions. Come on; let's learn some more.

> *Unless we put medical freedom into the Constitution, the time will come when medicine will organize into an undercover dictatorship to restrict the art of healing to one class of men and deny equal privileges to others: the Constitution of the Republic should make a special privilege for medical freedoms as well as religious freedom.*
>
> Benjamin Rush, MD
> (1745–1813)
>
> A signer of the Declaration of Independence
> and personal physician to George Washington

3

FREEDOM FROM PERIPHERAL NEUROPATHY

"The eye sees only what the mind is prepared to comprehend."

Henri Bergson

(1859 -1941)

Comprehension Is The Key To Recovery

Understanding neuropathy is the first step to gaining freedom from this condition. It is important that you have a basic comprehension of how this condition developed and how your nerves became damaged, so that once you've conquered this illness, you will not become afflicted with it again. This chapter will help you understand how your condition came to be and help you understand the bizarre symptoms. Later, in chapter 5, we will cover the specific causes of neuropathy.

Peripheral neuropathy is a term used to describe when the nerves outside of the brain and spinal cord, called peripheral nerves, have been damaged. These nerves are part of the vast communications network that transmits information from the brain and spinal cord, also known as the central nervous system (CNS), to every other part of your body. This damage can cause pain, numbness, tingling, and muscle weakness in the extremities. It usually affects the feet and legs, although the hands and arms can be affected, as well as organ systems.

Peripheral neuropathy comes in a few different forms, ranging from mononeuropathy, which is quite common, to polyneuropathy, which can be more serious in many cases because of the wider range of afflicted areas.

In mononeuropathy, only one nerve is affected, making it easier to diagnose. A common example of mononeuropathy includes carpal tunnel syndrome, in which the median nerve, which travels through the carpal tunnel of the wrist, becomes compressed. This is known as a repetitive strain injury and is a common occurrence in people who overuse computers. The pins-and-needles sensation of one's arm or leg falling asleep is caused by compression mononeuropathy. We refer to this sensation as a paresthesia, though this is a much less severe problem that is correctable by simply adjusting your body position.

Peripheral neuropathy might also be referred to as polyneuropathy. The term *polyneuropathy* is Greek in origin. *Poly* means "many." *Neuro* refers to nerves. *Pathy* refers to a disease. Therefore, polyneuropathy is a neurological disorder that occurs when many nerves throughout the body malfunction simultaneously. It might appear without warning, or it could develop gradually over a longer period of time. Peripheral neuropathy disorders are often symmetrical, affecting both of the feet and the hands, causing weakness, loss of sensation, pins-and-needle sensations, or burning pain.[6] In this regard, it is very different from mononeuropathy, which only affects one nerve.

Polyneuropathy has far-reaching and much more serious consequences. There are numerous conditions that can cause polyneuropathy; we will cover these in more depth later in the book. Although the different terms (peripheral neuropathy or polyneuropathy) are used interchangeably, the meaning remains the same. Damage has occurred to some part or parts of the nerves outside of your brain and spinal cord.

To fully understand your condition, I need to provide you with some basic information about your nervous system. Don't worry. It's not my intention to turn you into a neurologist. I merely want you to have a general understanding of your condition and its effects on your body.

ANATOMY OF A NERVE – *simplified*

Your nervous system is made up of two parts:

I. The central nervous system (CNS) includes the brain and the spinal cord.
II. The peripheral nervous system (PNS) connects the nerves running from the brain and spinal cord to the rest of the body—your arms, hands, legs, feet, internal organs, joints, mouth, eyes, ears, nose, and skin.

To understand how neuropathy occurs, let's look at the anatomy of a nerve.

Every nerve is made up of an axon, a myelin sheath, and a dendrite. Dendrites are long extensions that act like antennae so that one nerve can reach the next nerve. The job of a dendrite is to receive signals from the brain and spinal cord and then send that message down the nerve. An axon (a long slender projection of nerve cells) is your actual nerve fiber, which transmits information to all other cells of the body. Every healthy nerve is covered by a myelin sheath, a protective coating around the nerve that prevents interferences from occurring in the nerve signals. Aside from serving as a protective barrier, the myelin sheath also allows signal transmissions to occur unimpeded, and at a much faster rate, down the length of the nerve.

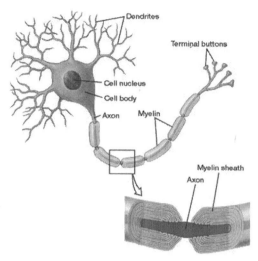

In order to help you visualize how your nerves function, imagine your landline telephone system. You have wire cables encased in rubber or plastic tubing. The wires in your telephone cable allow the transmission of messages from your location out to the world, much like the nerves in your body. The plastic tubing protects these wires from damage and also prevents external interference. This plastic tubing would be similar to the myelin sheath around your nerves.

Key constituents that make up the protective coating of myelin around nerves are fats—which make up 75 percent of the myelin—and proteins. This is important to know because many common medications, such as statin drugs

> Demyelination is similar to electrical wires without the rubber or plastic exterior around the wires, resulting in cross talk between nerves. This cross talk mimics static noise on a phone.

(cholesterol drugs), cause a breakdown in the fat of the myelin, damaging the protective coating of the nerve. We will discuss this in greater detail later. For now, what's important to know is that damage to the myelin sheath, also called demyelination, will cause signal impulses traveling along the nerve to slow down and possibly pick up interference—or static—along the way.

A. NORMAL HEALTHY NERVE
B. DAMAGE TO AXON
C. DAMAGE TO MYELIN SHEATH

Peripheral neuropathy occurs when damage is done to the nerve (axon), the protective coating (myelin sheath), or both of them. It can also occur when the gap between two nerves becomes too wide.

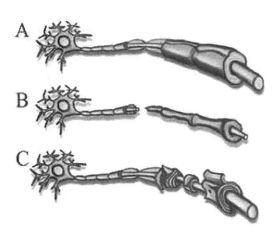

This damage can occur as a result of taking various medications or having conditions like diabetes or other metabolic disorders. When these nerves are damaged or destroyed, the nerves are prevented from sending messages from the brain and the spinal cord to the muscles, skin, and other parts of the body. Like static on a telephone line, peripheral neuropathy distorts and sometimes interrupts messages between the brain and the rest of the body.

In the most common forms of peripheral neuropathy, the nerve fibers that are farthest from the brain and the spinal cord malfunction first. This is why the most common point of origin for this disorder is the feet. Pain and other symptoms usually appear in a symmetrical distribution; for example, pain can start in both feet and gradually progress up both legs. As the condition advances, the fingers, hands, and arms may later become affected. With increasing severity and time, the condition can even progress into the central part, or trunk, of the body. It's very common for diabetics suffering from neuropathy to experience this pattern of ascending nerve damage.

TYPES OF NEUROPATHY

There are three types of peripheral nerves: motor, sensory, and autonomic. Some neuropathies affect all three types of nerves, while others may affect only one or two.

3 Types of Peripheral Nerves:
- Motor
- Sensory
- Autonomic

Motor nerves send impulses from the brain and the spinal cord to all of the muscles in the body. This permits people to do activities like walking, catching a ball, or moving the fingers to pick up objects. Motor nerve damage can lead to muscle weakness, difficulty walking and moving the arms, cramps, and spasms in the muscles.

Sensory nerves send messages from the muscles back to the spinal cord and the brain. Special sensors in the skin and deep inside the body help people identify whether an object is sharp or dull, hot or cold, or whether a body part is still or in motion. These nerve fibers allow us to feel pain. Sensory nerve damage often results in tingling, numbness, pain, and extreme sensitivity to touch.

<u>Autonomic nerves</u> control involuntary or semivoluntary functions such as heart rate, blood pressure, digestion, sweating, breathing and blinking. When the autonomic nerves are damaged, a person's heart might beat more quickly or slowly. These people might get dizzy when standing up, and they might sweat excessively or not at all. In addition, autonomic nerve damage might result in difficulty swallowing, nausea, vomiting, diarrhea, or constipation. Problems with urination, incontinence, abnormal pupil size, and sexual dysfunction may also result.

Peripheral nerve fibers can be classified according to size, which is determined by the thickness of the protective coating (myelin) around the nerve.

- **Large nerve fibers**—heavily myelinated, these fibers control motor strength, vibratory sensation, and touch sensation.
- **Small nerve fibers**—these contain both myelinated and unmyelinated fibers. They are responsible for innervating skin and involuntary muscles, including organ muscles such as the cardiac muscle, and smooth muscles like the kidney and liver. These fibers control pain sensation, temperature sensation, and autonomic functions.

The large fibers of the peripheral nerves, found within the motor fiber, are heavily myelinated to allow for very fast signal transmission to the muscles. Damage to these fibers will affect the muscles' ability to contract, resulting in loss of strength, muscular twitching, cramping, and spasms within the muscle. A person's sense of vibration and touch can also be affected, resulting in a loss of balance and coordination. Large nerve fibers are damaged at a slower rate than small nerve fibers.

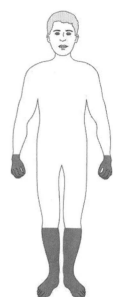

Small fiber neuropathy can involve damage to the nerves in the skin and organs; the damage can cause symptoms such as numbness, burning pain, deep-aching pain, pins-and-needles sensations, electrical shock-like sensations, or stabbing pain. This can result in an extreme sensitivity to light touch, making it unbearable for a person to tolerate the pressure of a bed sheet on their feet or legs. They can become sensitive enough that even the pressure of clothing against their skin can be intolerable.

Small nerve fiber damage in peripheral neuropathy initially begins with symptoms occurring in both feet, often in the soles. As the condition worsens, these symptoms spread up the leg. Typically, as the nerves at the calf level are damaged, the hands begin to show signs of nerve damage as well, and will display some of the same symptoms (burning, numbness, tingling, aching, or stabbing pain). Since these symptoms will occur over the region of the feet and legs that socks would cover, and over the areas of the hand that a glove would cover, it is known as the **stocking and glove** distribution.

These patients typically report that their symptoms worsen at night. This occurs because there are fewer distractions to the nervous system. When a person is in bed, lying down, waiting for sleep, there is less input to the nervous system (i.e., less information that the nervous system has to process). As a result, the nervous system's focus and attention is concentrated on the dysfunction of the peripheral nerves.

Autonomic neuropathy is a form of polyneuropathy that affects the part of the nervous system that is under involuntary control. The autonomic nervous system affects mostly the internal organs, such as the bladder muscles, the cardiovascular system, the digestive tract, and the genital organs. These nerves are not under a person's conscious control; they function automatically. For instance, a healthy heart at rest will beat between sixty and ninety times per minute. This is not something that you need to think about for it to occur. The body is automatically programmed to maintain your heartbeat. You also do not need to think about taking a breath or digesting your food. These are all autonomic nerve functions.

Damage to the small nerve fibers of the autonomic system is more common than most people realize. An affected person can develop swelling, temperature changes, or color changes in their feet from vascular impairment. One of my patients felt as if her feet were on fire, as a result. The burning would become so intense that she would soak her feet in an ice bath for fifteen to twenty minutes to get relief.

A person may also experience changes in the texture of the skin on their legs from this type of nerve damage. Their skin can become extremely thin and shiny. Once the small nerve fibers are damaged, the skin cells no longer receive stimulation from the nervous system signaling them to produce new skin cells. Without new skin cell production, the old skin cells reach maturity and die off, resulting in thin, shiny skin.

When the damage to the autonomic small nerve fibers has become widespread, internal organ dysfunction can occur. It may manifest as dysfunction in GI (gastrointestinal) motility resulting in either diarrhea or constipation. A person might also suffer from mild to severe bowel or bladder incontinence and even erectile dysfunction (ED). Small nerve fiber damage can also cause blood pressure irregularities or heart palpitations.

By far, the most common type of peripheral neuropathy is sensorimotor neuropathy, in which both the sensory and the motor nerve fibers are damaged or destroyed. There are many causes of sensorimotor neuropathy, which we will later discuss in greater detail.

SYMPTOMS OF NEUROPATHY

Neuropathy can have many different symptoms, depending on which group or groups of nerves are involved (motor, sensory, or autonomic). Previously, I mentioned that the most common forms of neuropathy include both motor and sensory nerves. Symptoms that commonly result from this include:

- Muscle weakness
- Muscle loss
- Inability to grasp objects
- Painful cramps or muscle twitching
- Numbness and tingling

- Burning sensation
- Extreme sensitivity to touch or pressure
- Sharp, stabbing or lightning bolt pain
- Lack of balance, and coordination
- Bone degeneration
- Unusual sweating or complete inability to sweat
- Changes in skin, hair, and nails
- Abnormalities in blood pressure, heart rate or pulse
- Sensation of wearing a glove or stocking.

Peripheral neuropathy usually starts with numbness, prickling, or tingling in the toes or fingers. It might spread up the feet to the legs, or it might affect the hands with gradual damage spanning up the arms. Damage can cause burning, freezing, throbbing, or shooting pain that is often worse at night.

The pain can be either constant or periodic, but usually the pain is felt equally on both sides of the body—in both hands or in both feet. Some types of peripheral neuropathy develop suddenly, while others progress more slowly over many years.

Often, people suffering from peripheral neuropathy will lose their balance and coordination because of the loss of specialized receptors located on nerve endings found in muscles, tendons, joints, and the inner ear. These receptors are called proprioceptors, but to keep it simple we will simply refer to them as receptors. The job of these receptors is to relay information about our motion or position. It allows us to control our limbs without directly looking at them. For example, you can walk in a straight line without looking down at your feet, and you can touch your nose with your finger while your eyes are closed. These same receptors are partly responsible for our balance and coordination. One of the most common complaints I hear from patients suffering from neuropathy is that they feel unstable, and they tend to fall. This is very frustrating and embarrassing for them—not to mention dangerous.

Falls are the leading cause of death among the elderly. Eighty-seven percent of all fractures in the elderly are due to falls. One out of five seniors will die within five years following a hip fracture. A loss of balance is major risk factor for neuropathy sufferers.

4

SHOCKING FACTS ABOUT YOUR MEDICATIONS AND NEUROPATHY

"It is easy to get a thousand prescriptions but hard to get one single remedy."

~Chinese Proverb~

Blood Pressure Medications and Insanity

One in three adults suffers from high blood pressure, as reported by the CDC in 2011—approximately sixty-eight million people in the United States. Blood pressure is the force of blood against your artery walls as it circulates through your body. Blood pressure normally rises and falls throughout the day, but it can cause health problems if it stays elevated for a long time.

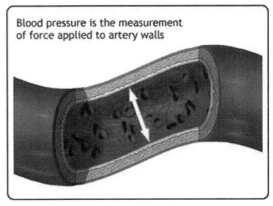

Blood pressure is the measurement of force applied to artery walls

It astounds me that hypertension (high blood pressure) is treated as a disease in this country. It is not a disease; it is a symptom of a dysfunction within the body. Imagine that one day, as you are driving to work, the engine light suddenly comes on in the dashboard of your car. You do the responsible thing that any car owner would do; you ignore it for a week or two in hopes it will disappear. When it doesn't turn off after two weeks, you finally take it to your mechanic. He pops the hood, looks underneath it, and states, "I know exactly what the problem is, and I can fix it for you." He takes a pair of wire cutters and cuts the wire to the engine light and—poof, presto, magic—the engine light goes off. Now, I ask you, did this fix the problem? Of course not. However, every day this is how we address our issues with blood pressure—by taking medications that cover up the real reason behind the elevation in our blood pressure. Instead, we need to identify the problem that is causing our blood pressure to elevate, and then fix that. Treating only the symptom can have dire consequences.

A survey published in the *British Medical Journal* found that 97 percent of patients taking blood pressure medications suffered from significant side effects, including neuropathy.

One known side effect of blood pressure medication is the damage that can occur at the nerve sites for a variety of reasons, ranging from decreased blood flow at the feet or hands—to disruption in nerve transmission due to mineral loss or depletion.

High blood pressure medication not only lowers blood pressure; it also reduces the ability of the arterial blood to refill the vessels. This creates a tendency for the blood to pool in the

> *Neuropathy is a prevalent side effect caused by many blood pressure medications.*

lower extremities. As a result, the nerves and their junctions, called synaptic junctions, do not have enough of the nutrients and oxygen necessary to maintain their health, leading to nerve cell atrophy, loss of mineralization, and decreased conductivity of the nerve at the synaptic junctions.

First, let's address the role that decreased blood flow plays in the health of your nerves. Diminished blood flow to the hands or feet means diminished oxygenation to the tissues, including the nerves. To survive in this oxygen-depleted environment, the nerve cells can temporarily contract or shrink (atrophy) to conserve oxygen and stay alive. Each nerve cell is separated from the adjacent cell by a gap called the synaptic junction. The shrinkage of each nerve cell due to lack of oxygen can increase this gap, enlarging the synaptic junction. These junctions do not come into contact with each other, and as a result, nerve impulses must jump across this gap.

A larger gap makes it harder for the electrical nerve impulse to get across. When the gap gets too big, the electrical impulse can't make the transition across this gap. This means that the message being delivered along the nerve never makes it to its destination or is misdirected to a different part of the body; it will then be misinterpreted as pain. At times, the nerve signals may begin to pile up on one side of the gap until they can make it across to the other side. Once a collection of these signals gets large enough, a very large signal can be pushed across the widened gap. When this occurs, the brain will interpret it as a sharp, stabbing, or shooting pain. This is what is referred to as impaired nerve function.

We must also realize that once this gap inhibits peripheral nerve impulses, the minerals that are dissolved in the synaptic junction's fluid, such as calcium, can leach out, making the fluid less conductive. Water alone does not conduct electricity. Water needs minerals dissolved in it to make it conductive. A wider gap equals a loss of minerals and therefore loss of conductivity.

Beta Blockers

Some of the most commonly prescribed blood pressure medications are beta blockers. Beta blockers block the effects of the hormones norepinephrine and epinephrine, also known as adrenaline. This occurs by blocking beta receptor sites on the cell. When you take beta blockers, blood vessels narrow and constrict, allowing the heart to beat more slowly and with less force, thereby reducing blood pressure. The narrowing of blood vessels also causes a decrease in blood flow to tissues. Any decrease in blood flow will result in anoxia; so many tissues will be deprived of necessary oxygen and nutrients.

This affects tissues that are the farthest away—especially the feet and the legs—potentially leading to peripheral nerve damage.

A further problem of using beta blockers is that beta receptor sites are not isolated to the heart. They are also located on other organs, including the pancreas, liver,

Number of Prescriptions filled in 2010

191.5 million scripts for beta blockers

87.4 million scripts for ACE inhibitors

57.2 million calcium channel blockers

ARBs accounted for $7 billion in sales in 2010

lungs, and kidneys. Any beta blocker that is not cardio-selective will affect receptor sites outside of the heart and this can create a narrowing of these arteries. As a result, **beta blockers have been linked with an increased risk for developing diabetes**. As reported in the *American Journal of Cardiology* in 2007, a meta-analysis of 94,492 patients taking beta blockers resulted in a 22 percent increased risk for new-onset diabetes. As you will recall, diabetes and peripheral neuropathy go hand in hand, with 60 to 70 percent of diabetics developing neuropathy. **This same study also revealed that beta blocker usage resulted in a 15 percent increased risk for stroke.**

Another harmful effect commonly associated with the use of these drugs is that they can actually worsen respiratory diseases, including asthma, by constricting the blood vessels in the lungs and narrowing the walls of the airways. On top of all of this, beta blockers have also been known to worsen preexisting heart conditions, according to the *Drug Information Handbook, 15th edition*. Examples of beta blockers include acebutolol (Sectral), atenolol (Tenormin), bisoprolol (Zebeta), metoprolol (Lopressor, Toprol-XL), nadolol (Corgard), nebivolol (Bystolic), and propranolol (Inderal, **Inderal LA**). Did you know that **191.5 million prescriptions** were filled in 2010 alone?

ACE Inhibitors

Another common blood pressure medication falls into a class called ACE Inhibitors (angiotensin converting enzyme). ACE Inhibitors relax blood vessels by preventing an enzyme in your body from producing angiotensin II. This inhibition of angiotensin II affects blood vessels of the heart, and it has an impact on other organs, such as the kidneys, the lungs, and also on hormones.

For instance, although these drugs preserve the function of the kidneys in people with diabetes whose kidneys are normal, they can be very dangerous for people who have kidneys that are damaged or poorly functioning. In extreme cases, ACE inhibitors have actually been associated with kidney damage. When a person suffers from kidney disease, toxins begin to build up in the bloodstream. These toxins have damaging effects on peripheral nerves. Other unfortunate side effects of ACE inhibitors are that they can reduce the moisture in a person's lungs and thereby increase the risk of respiratory infection. They can also cause a nonproductive chronic cough. This side effect is quite commonly experienced by a large number of people who have taken ACE inhibitors. ACE inhibitors have also been known to cause elevated blood potassium levels, a condition referred to as hypokalemia. Potassium is an important electrolyte found both inside and outside of cells. Potassium regulates heart rate and rhythm, and it also controls both muscle and nerve functions. Elevated levels of potassium not only can be life-threatening by stopping regular cardiac function, but can also prevent normal nerve firing. **Elevated potassium suppresses the nerve from firing its message.** In the beginning, this might manifest with typical neuropathy symptoms; however, over time this can result in a general paralysis of skeletal muscles.

Several examples of ACE inhibitors are benazepril (Lotensin), captopril, enalapril (Vasotec), fosinopril, lisinopril (Prinivil, Zestril), moexipril (Univasc), perindopril (Aceon), quinapril (Accupril), ramipril (Altace), trandolapril (Mavik). Take note that <u>87.4 million scripts</u> are written, per year, for lisinopril alone.

Calcium Channel Blockers

Calcium channel blockers, also known as CCBs, are **the most toxic class of blood pressure medications**. They are widely prescribed in the US for conditions such as hypertension (high blood pressure), heart arrhythmias (irregular heartbeats), and angina (chest pains). The use of CCBs has been associated with a large number of harmful side effects, including peripheral neuropathy. Let's take a look at how this occurs.

We're familiar with the role that calcium plays in healthy teeth and bones, but did you know that it is also required for healthy functioning of every cell in your body? It aids in constricting and relaxing blood vessels. It plays a role in the secretion of hormones, like insulin, for example. Calcium is also used for nerve impulse transmission (moving a signal along nerve pathways) and muscle contractions. For the purpose of this book, we are going to focus on calcium's role in nerve transmissions.

Cells, such as skeletal muscles and nerve cells, contain calcium channels in their cell membranes. These channels open and close to allow for rapid changes in calcium concentrations. For example, a muscle fiber will receive a nerve impulse (signal) that stimulates it to contract. When this occurs, calcium channels in the cell membrane open to allow a few calcium molecules into the muscle cell. These molecules bind to activator proteins within the cell, releasing a flood of calcium from storage sites inside the cell. The binding of calcium to the protein initiates a series of steps that lead to muscle contractions.

When calcium is not present in sufficient amounts, cellular membranes become irritable, which can lead to muscle spasms that manifest as tremors or muscle cramps. As you will recall, I promised that I would not attempt to turn you into a neurologist, so this is a very simplified version of how calcium affects nerve cells. I have left out quite a few intermediate steps, but I have supplied you with the overall meat and potatoes for you to get the gist.

Dangers of CCBs

1. Increases risk of heart attack by 60 percent
2. Increases risk of cancer
3. Increases risk of developing depression or anxiety
4. Commonly leads to peripheral neuropathy
5. Can cause GI disorders

Calcium channel blocker medications disrupt the action of these calcium channels. As a result, they interfere with the flow of calcium and impair nerve function. It is possible for nerves to heal from the damage done to their calcium channels, but it can take anywhere from months to years for this to occur.

CCBs such as Cardizem, Adalat, and Procardia lower blood pressure by blocking the entrance of calcium into the arterial wall cells. This causes the vessels to become more relaxed and less constricted. As a result of blocking calcium channels into a cell, over time the calcium channel will stop functioning altogether. Initially, symptoms of high blood pressure or chest pains may improve, but later on, these drugs poison the channels so badly that they are known to cause many terrible symptoms, including heart failure, increased risk of cancer, and early death. In the winter of 1996, the highly acclaimed *Wall Street Journal* reported that patients who took calcium channel blockers had a 60 percent increased chance of dying of a heart attack based on a study performed by Bruce Psaty, MD.

In the *Clinical Pharmacy Review*, Susan Ross, MD, states, "Calcium is an essential component in a variety of cardiovascular functions. The contractile processes of the heart and smooth muscle, the initiation of action potentials in cardiac conducting cells, and the storage and use of energy in the myocardium *(heart wall)* are all dependent upon the presence of calcium." She goes on to say, "Therefore, calcium blockers accomplish the desired effect of lowering high blood pressure by blocking the essential functions of the heart and blood vessel cells." She is articulating that this is a very ineffective—not to mention dangerous—way to lower blood pressure. It is not what we would call a good trade-off; you lower your blood pressure only to set the stage for other chronic illnesses to take hold down the line due to the calcium disruption that these medications (CCBs) have caused.

This information is nothing new. In the medical community, we have known for a long time that calcium is essential to heart function.

> **CALCIUM REDUCES HYPERTENSION**
>
> Daily calcium intake of 1,000–1,200 mg/day reduced blood pressure significantly.
>
> DASH STUDY

The relationship between calcium intake and blood pressure has been investigated extensively over the past two decades. An analysis of twenty-three large observational studies found a reduction in systolic and diastolic blood pressure when calcium was consumed daily. In these studies, calcium supplementation ranged from 500–2,000 mg/day, with 1,000–1,500 mg/day being the most common dose. Furthermore, in the DASH (Dietary Approaches to Stop

Hypertension) study, 549 people were randomized to one of three diets for eight weeks:

(1) A control diet that was **low** in fruit, vegetables, and dairy products.
(2) A diet **rich** in fruits (~5 servings/day) and vegetables (~3 servings/day).
(3) A **combination diet** that was rich in fruits and vegetables, as well as low-fat dairy products (~3 servings/day).

The combination diet delivered 800 mg more calcium per day over the control diet and fruit/vegetable-rich diets, for a total of about 1,200 mg of calcium/day. Among those participants diagnosed with hypertension, the combination diet reduced systolic blood pressure by 11.4 mm Hg and diastolic pressure by 5.5 mm Hg more than the control diet.

This research indicates that a calcium intake at the recommended level (1,000-1,200 mg/day) may be helpful in preventing and treating moderate hypertension. More information about the DASH diet is available from the National Institutes of Health (NIH).

One can clearly see that blocking the flow of calcium is dangerous, since calcium is essential for normal cell life and operation. Without sufficient calcium, you can't survive. Calcium channel blockers have been linked to contributing to or creating neuropathies. Many previous studies have associated calcium channel blockers with increased risks of heart attacks, breast cancer, and suicide, as well as increased gastrointestinal bleeding. The *American Journal of Hypertension* published a research article showing a correlation between taking calcium channel blockers and increased risk of cancer. In August 2000, a report from the meeting of the European Society of Cardiology in Amsterdam (Netherlands) showed that despite lowering blood pressure, calcium channel blockers did not reduce the death rate. An astounding 57.2 million prescriptions of Norvasc, a popular CCB, were written in one year; and that's simply one out of many prescriptions written for a number of CCBs.

Angiotensin Receptor Blockers

The last class of blood pressure medications is the ARBs or angiotensin receptor blockers.

Angiotensin II receptor blockers inhibit a substance that normally would cause blood vessels to narrow or constrict. As a result of this inhibition, blood vessels relax and widen. This dilation allows the blood to flow easily through the vessels. This in turn reduces blood pressure. The problem with ARBs is that they increase the release of water and sodium into the urine, and they act directly on the hormones that regulate sodium and water balance. Sodium is an electrolyte, which means that it has an electrical charge. Sodium helps control the functioning of nerves and muscles, and it is also important for regulating pressure. Your body needs sodium in certain amounts to function properly. If your sodium levels get too low, you have a condition known as hyponatremia.

> ARB medications can increase your risk for heart attacks.
>
> *Journal of the American Heart Association*

Hyponatremia can cause neurological problems and permanent nerve damage. Acute hyponatremia must be treated carefully, as improper treatment can make the nerve damage worse. Sodium levels can decrease within the body due to medications like ARBs and diuretics. When the sodium levels in your blood get too low, water travels into your cells to help balance the sodium levels. This causes the cells to swell, which can result in nerve damage, also known as neuropathy.

ARBs are prescribed to decrease blood pressure and also to decrease cardiovascular incidences and myocardial infarctions (heart attacks). Ironically, according to an article in the *Journal of the American Heart Association* titled "Circulation," **ARB medications were actually found to increase the risk of myocardial infarction.** These medications accounted for $7 billion worth of sales alone in 2010.

A few of the names of ARB medications are Advent, candesartan (Atacand), eprosartan (Teveten), irbesartan (Avapro), losartan (Cozaar), olmesartan (Benicar), telmisartan (Micardis), and valsartan (Diovan).

As alarming as this information is, I am in no way advocating that a person should abruptly discontinue their medication. It's extremely important for anyone currently taking any of these medications to realize that *you should never abruptly stop taking your blood pressure medication—or any medication,* for that matter. **Discontinuing your medication suddenly might put you at serious health risk, and it might even jeopardize your life.** Any medication must be gradually tapered off under your doctor's supervision.

Cholesterol Medications:

What the pharmaceutical companies don't want you to know...

Cholesterol lowering drugs are the most commonly prescribed types of medication in the United States. , These prescriptions are handed out like candy with blatant disregard for what caused the cholesterol levels to elevate in the first place. In all, more than 255 *million* prescriptions were dispensed for these drugs in 2010.

The most widely prescribed cholesterol-reducing medications are a group of drugs called *statins*. They are drugs like Advicor, Altoprev, Crestor, Lipitor, Simcor, Vytorin, and Zocor. Statin drugs are now prescribed to over thirteen million Americans and are responsible for generating over $20 billion in revenue in this country alone. In fact, spending on cholesterol-lowering drugs like statins increased by $160 million in 2010, as reported by the IMS Institute for Healthcare Informatics article, "Use of Medicines in the United States: Review of 2010."

> **FDA DEMANDS WARNING LABEL FOR STATIN DRUGS**
>
> *Warning! Statin drugs can cause the following:*
>
> - **Diabetes**
> - **Liver damage**
> - **Memory loss and confusion**
> - **Muscle weakness and atrophy** (certain statins).

It's widely published in the research that the same statin drugs that reduce cholesterol can cause peripheral neuropathy—damage to the nerves in your feet, legs, hands, and arms.

Statin drugs are very good at blocking cholesterol production in the liver—so good, in fact, that they can cause nerve degeneration or breakdown. As you will recall, a protective coating called the myelin sheath surrounds nerve cells. This sheath is made up of protein and fat (cholesterol).

When you take a statin drug, otherwise known as a cholesterol-inhibiting drug, this can cause a breakdown of the fat in the myelin sheath around the nerve. This breakdown is called demyelination of the nerve, which leads to significant nerve injury.

A researcher from Denmark, David Gaist, MD, was one of the first to report the link between statin drugs and nerve injury. His study was published in the journal Neurology in 2002. His research revealed that people taking statin drugs had a **16:1-fold increased risk** *of developing neuropathy* compared to people not taking statins. Furthermore, people who had taken statins for two or more years had **26.4 times more risk of developing neuropathy**. When taking a larger dose of the drug, the risk increased. (*Neurology,* 2002; 58; 1333-1337.) The study is summarized on the website for the American Academy of Neurology.

Research performed at Fukui Medical University in Fukui, Japan, revealed that simvastatin (Zocor) had neurotoxic effects on peripheral nerves, resulting in nerve dysfunction in some cases and nerve death in others. This type of nerve damage is what's called direct nerve damage. The drug directly affects the nerve, leading to injury and damage—and thus, polyneuropathy. Let's also take a look at how statin drugs create indirect damage to the peripheral nerves.

A new study, recently released by the Women's Health Initiative and published in the *Archives of Internal Medicine* in 2012, confirms a dangerous statin drug side effect: diabetes. Researchers at Harvard Medical School report that women over the age of forty-five are much more likely to develop diabetes if they're taking a statin drug. This information is hardly new to us. There have been several studies that reported the same findings. ***Statin use has been linked to increased inci-***

dence of type II diabetes. Statins have been on the market since the 1980s but it has taken twenty years for a number of their dangerous side effects to surface, as is typical with most medications. In January 2008, a study was published in the journal *Diabetes*. **This study revealed that statin drugs increased insulin resistance.** Don't forget, first comes insulin resistance, next comes diabetes. Later in 2011, findings were published in *JAMA* revealing that people taking high-dose statins were 12 percent more likely to get diabetes. As all of the evidence was compiling at an astronomical rate, the FDA finally decided to speak out, though they were careful not to offend the pharmaceutical companies.

> **DANGERS OF USING STATIN DRUGS**
> 1. Peripheral Neuropathy
> 2. Muscle weakness and atrophy
> 3. Developing Diabetes
> 4. Memory loss
> 5. Impaired vitamin D function
> 6. Impaired sex hormone function
> 7. Depletes Co Q-10
> 8. Increases cancer risk
> 9. Birth defects

The US Food and Drug Administration (FDA) has issued new labeling guidelines for statin drugs warning users that the medications can cause memory loss, elevated blood sugar levels, and type 2 diabetes, in addition to muscle damage and liver disease. On its website the FDA writes, "The reports about memory loss, forgetfulness, and confusion span all statin products and all age groups," and "raised blood sugar levels and the development of type 2 diabetes have been reported with the use of statins." More than twenty million Americans are currently taking statin drugs. When looking at the percentages, that equates to approximately one hundred thousand new cases of diabetes as a result of statin use. As you will recall, diabetes indirectly causes peripheral neuropathy by wreaking havoc with circulation, not to mention the damage that excess glucose in the bloodstream causes to neurons.

Still, US doctors have tended to discount these findings, says David Perlmutter, MD, a neurologist, fellow of the American College of Nutrition, and director of the Perlmutter Health Center, in Naples, Florida. "These drugs are big money-makers, and many doctors turn a blind eye to things they do not want to see," he says. "These drugs are supposed to be used only after strict diet and lifestyle recommendations have failed, but in this country, the whole message about diet and exercise has been lost and we are paying the price for it. We have medical offices filled with patients with muscle and nerve damage from statin drugs." And when nerves are damaged, Dr. Perlmutter says, "it can be very challenging to heal the situation." It can take a year or even longer to see improvement, but it can happen.

Most people have been pounded down by their family doctors, who try to fill them with fear if they even consider not taking a cholesterol medication. One well-meaning—albeit ignorant—doctor told one of my patients that she was going to die if she didn't take her statin drug. That was actually what this doctor said. You have been told for decades that if you do not control your cholesterol, the chances are high that you will suffer a stroke or a heart attack. Because of this, I watch people fight to get to the front of the line to receive their statin drugs. In response to possibly getting off of them, many of them exclaim, "Are you insane?"

In fact, I was treating a nurse for disc problems. She would, faithfully, have biannual blood work performed to monitor her health levels, and would always furnish me with a copy of her lab results. I noticed that her blood work was fantastic, yet she was taking a statin drug, so I asked her why. She replied, "Oh, heart disease is rampant in my family and several years ago my cholesterol was slightly elevated, so my family doctor placed me on it." Based on the current research showing all of the damaging effects caused by statins, I would not have been in agreement with her *ever* going on any statin drug. However, I respectfully said to her, "OK. But your lab work for the past year has shown perfect cholesterol levels, so why are you still taking this drug?" She confided in me that she had raised this question to her medical doctor, who told her that she needed to stay on the drug as a precautionary measure. He also told her that if she *ever* were to go off this medication, given her family history, she would run an extremely high risk of suffering a stroke or heart attack. As you can imagine, there's no way on this green earth she would even consider going off her statin. I was flabbergasted and disgusted by this doctor's ignorance, so I began to educate my patient. I provided her with untainted and unbiased research on statin drugs. She was dumbfounded. She asked me, "How come my doctor doesn't know about this?" What I really wanted to say—out of frustration from closed-minded, ill-informed doctors—was, "Probably because he's too damn lazy to research it." You will be pleased to know, though, that I held my tongue and gave her the politically correct answer. I said, "He's probably just unaware of the latest research." Since she had been a nurse for twenty-five years, she decided to wean herself off her statin drug. She has now been off them for two years, and her cholesterol is great. Incidentally, she noticed after getting off the statin, she no longer suffered from daily muscle pain and weakness. She had never realized that her symptoms were side effects of the statin medication.

So– how could a person ever consider discontinuing their statin drug, even if it was contributing to or causing their neuropathy? First, you must become accurately informed of the research findings—that is, studies that have not been funded by the same pharmaceutical companies that are making multibillions of dollars in profits selling these medications. Let's begin by understanding the role that cholesterol plays in the body.

Cholesterol is a specialized type of lipid that is known as a sterol, and it is produced in the liver. Body fat or dietary fat, on the other hand, are from glyceryl esters. We won't delve too deeply into this. The key to remember is that dietary cholesterol is not the same cholesterol that is produced in the liver. The cholesterol levels measured on blood work are representative of liver function– not what you've consumed in your diet.

Elevated cholesterol is a symptom of an underlying health problem and nothing more. It is not a disease in itself. Cholesterol is simply the messenger that lets us know that there is abnormal or prolonged stress on the liver. It is not the enemy. Research shows that elevated cholesterol is a poor predictor for strokes or heart attacks. Elevated cholesterol levels predict less than 35 percent of cardiovascular diseases. In fact, research indicates that most heart attacks and strokes occur in individuals with normal cholesterol levels.

> Research reveals that elevated fasting insulin levels are a better predictor of cardiovascular disease than cholesterol levels.

Did you know that insulin controls the production of fats, such as cholesterol and triglycerides? It also controls the packaging of cholesterol and triglycerides into LDL (low-density lipoproteins), VLDL (very low-density lipoproteins), HDL (high-density lipoproteins), and other lipoproteins. When your insulin levels are higher, also known as insulin resistance, so is your cholesterol production. **One very effective way to decrease cholesterol naturally is by decreasing insulin levels and making your cells more sensitive to insulin.** When we consume sugar, processed carbohydrates, or alcohol (alcohol is converted into sugar in the body), we produce more insulin hormones.

This, in turn, stimulates more cholesterol and triglycerides to be produced. Therefore, people with type 2 diabetes have elevated fasting insulin (high insulin levels in the absence of a meal), as well as elevated cholesterol. In fact, numerous studies have indicated that elevated fasting insulin is a better predictor of cardiovascular disease than cholesterol. Research has also indicated that the best predictors of increased cardiovascular risk for stroke or heart attack are homocysteine and C-reactive protein (CRP). These are very simple tests that can be—but seldom are—ordered on your blood work lab panel.

Cholesterol is not the bad guy. In fact, it is essential for good health. There is not one single cell in your body that doesn't rely upon cholesterol for its healthy membrane structure. Cholesterol is an essential component of cell membranes, and it plays a critical role in cell communication. Without cholesterol, cell membranes lose their normal function. Cholesterol plays a vital role in both the PNS and CNS, and it has an essential role in the brain's structure and functioning. Cholesterol is also the foundational material of many essential enzymes, hormones, and vitamins, including vitamin D, steroid hormones, and the bile acids that are necessary for digestion. Recent studies have even shown that cholesterol might have protective properties against cancer.

A thirty-year study published in the Journal of the American Medical Association *provides evidence that elevated cholesterol in people over the age of fifty does not increase their risk of heart attack.*

Cholesterol levels were measured in people who did not have coronary heart disease (CHD) or cancer. The study found that there was no increase in the death rates of those with high cholesterol. Research also reveals that elevated cholesterol has protective effects and is not harmful to the elderly. A separate study published in the *European Heart Journal* in 1997 found that the risk of cardiac death was the same in groups of people with low or normal cholesterol levels as those with high cholesterol.

The source of this widespread confusion over whether statin drugs actually help reduce the risk of heart attacks or do more harm comes from the conflicting research. According to Dr. Peter Dingle, PhD, an environmental and nutritional toxicologist and an esteemed associate professor of health and the environment at Murdoch University, "Most of what we know about statins and their effects (beneficial or otherwise) actually comes directly from the scientific trials themselves, which were funded by, and even coordinated by, the drug companies. The vast majority of these studies were not from long-term, independent, evidence-based observations. As a result, all the information we have received is strongly biased." (8)

The major drug companies, as part of a marketing scheme, have become quite successful at convincing the public that lower cholesterol levels equal good health. Your family doctor, who has unwittingly become the retail arm or dispensary of the pharmaceutical industry, has aided these companies. How could your excellent, caring doctor allow this to happen? Most probably, they are not doing their homework. They are not reading the scientific literature—unbiased research that is not funded by the same drug company that is profiting from the sale of the drug it is promoting. Drug companies have convinced both the doctor and the public about the benefits of taking their drugs. Your doctors might also be relying upon the pharmaceutical reps to educate them. These pharmaceutical companies are not concerned about your good health; they are concerned about their profits. If everyone were to reclaim their health, the profits on Big Pharma would plunge.

> Antidepressants are the third most widely prescribed group of drugs in the US.

Antidepressants- The Epidemic

In this stressful, fast-paced, hectic world, Americans are popping more antidepressants than ever before. As revealed in one particular study, these drugs, once only prescribed by psychiatrists, are now being prescribed by family doctors, internal medicine doctors, neurologists, and cardiologists, to name a few, even in the absence of a mental health diagnosis, to treat normal daily stress. The Centers for Disease Control (CDC) reported on October 19, 2011, that 11 percent of Americans over the age of twelve take antidepressants. This was based on data in a study compiled by the National Center for Health Statistics. This means that slightly more than one out of ten people in the United States take antidepressant medication. We have seen an astronomical rise of 400 percent increased use of antidepressants since the first SSRI (selective serotonin reuptake inhibitor) hit the market in the 1980s. In fact, antidepressants like Lexapro, Paxil, and Prozac are now the third most widely prescribed group of drugs in the US.

So, what's the problem with using antidepressants, and how does this relate to neuropathy? A research study released by the **Diabetes Prevention Program Research Group revealed that continuous antidepressant use was significantly associated with an increased risk of developing diabetes.** This study found that it wasn't the depression that caused diabetes; it was the use of an antidepressant drug that correlated with the outcome of diabetes. Patients without diabetes who suffered from depression but did not use antidepressants did not develop diabetes. This is an astonishing finding, especially in light of the increased use of antidepressant medication among both teens and adults. In the section on diabetes, we discussed how neuropathy is indirectly caused by diabetes. In light of this study, it's no wonder that we are seeing ever-increasing cases of polyneuropathy develop with people using antidepressants.

> Antidepressant use has increased by 400 percent since the 1980s.

Common tricyclic antidepressants prescribed for neuropathy include: imipramine (Tofranil), amitriptyline (Elavil), and nortriptyline (Pamelor, Aventyl). Elavil is currently the most commonly prescribed antidepressant medication for peripheral neuropathy. This, by the way, is an off-label use of Elavil.

Another class of antidepressants, known as SSRIs (selective serotonin reuptake inhibitor) and SNRIs, (serotonin norepinephrine reuptake inhibitor) are commonly prescribed for treating chronic pain. Research studies from the Mayo Clinic have shown that, although these drugs help with some forms of chronic pain, they have minimal results with relieving neuropathic pain. Despite this research, there are still quite a few prescriptions written for SNRIs such as venlafaxine (Effexor) and duloxetine (Cymbalta), and SSRIs like paroxetine (Paxil) and fluoxetine (Prozac). Studies found that these drugs don't appear to help relieve pain on their own.

Over-The-Counter (OTC) Pain Killers

Millions of consumers turn to over-the-counter (OTC) pain medications daily to combat headaches, muscular aches, arthritis, colds, and fevers. The two most common types of OTC pain relievers used by both adults and children are NSAIDs, (nonsteroidal anti-inflammatory drugs)—such

PAIN RELIEVERS	
Bayer	Aleve
Bufferin	Naprosyn
Motrin	Tylenol
Advil	Excedrin

LINKED WITH PERIPHERAL NEUROPATHY

as aspirin, ibuprofen, and naproxen—and acetaminophen (Tylenol). NSAIDs help reduce the inflammation caused by injuries or arthritis. They are used to stop muscle aches and pains, headaches, and menstrual cramps. They are also used to reduce swelling and stiffness. Acetaminophen is used as a general pain reliever, and it is used for fever reduction.

OTC pain relievers are among the most widely used pain medications. According to a survey from the National Consumers League (NCL), 175 million Americans use them yearly, and they are a staple in every medicine cabinet around the country. Fortunately, they are completely safe—or are they? OTCs can be safe when used sparingly and when label directions are followed closely. Let me ask you: When was the last time you read the label on a bottle of Tylenol or Motrin that you have recently purchased? If you are like most people, you have not read this label. After all, Tylenol and Motrin cannot possibly harm you. If they could, they would not be easily accessible and sold over the counter, right? Guess again. The NCL reports that up to 16,500 people die each year from NSAID-related GI bleeding with an additional 107,000 people being hospitalized due to NSAID-related complications. The NCL further states that "a third of all consumers take more than the recommended dose of an OTC drug thinking it will increase the drug's effectiveness. But studies have linked overuse of anti-inflammatories and acetaminophen with kidney and liver problems." A study published in *Archives of Internal Medicine* found additional evidence of kidney damage when it discovered that men taking acetaminophen six or seven days a week had a 34 percent higher risk of hypertension. The risk for those who took NSAIDs for six or seven days per week was 38 percent higher and those who took aspirin six or

> Kidney and liver damage can cause polyneuropathy.

seven days per week was 26 percent higher. The cause for alarm with these statistics is that hypertension is often the very first sign of kidney disease, which has already been linked to the use of all common over-the-counter painkillers.

"Overuse of nonsteroidal anti-inflammatory drugs (NSAIDs), such as ibuprofen, aspirin, and naproxen, can cause bleeding ulcers, raise blood pressure, damage the esophagus, and lead to problems with the kidneys," says Jan Engle, PharmD, a pharmacist at the University Of Illinois College Of Pharmacy in Chicago and a past president of the American Pharmacists Association. According to the FDA, acetaminophen can be equally lethal. In fact, the overuse of this drug is one of the leading causes of liver failure in the United States. Data from both the FDA's Adverse Reporting System and the Acute Liver Failure Study Group showed reported that as little as 4g/day could lead to liver injury and consistent use of 7.5 g/day can lead to severe liver injury, as reported in the 2005 issue *Hepatology* by Anne M. Larson, MD and twenty-one colleagues. In 2007 a CDC report estimated that overdoses have resulted in more than 56,000 injuries, 26,000 hospitalizations, and an estimated 458 deaths per year.

Both kidney and liver damage can result in polyneuropathy. A research study done by the Department of Neurology at the Johns Hopkins University School of Medicine found that peripheral neuropathy has a strong association with chronic liver disease. In their study, they found that 71 percent of participants with chronic liver disease were found to have sensorimotor peripheral neuropathy, while an additional 48 percent of the patients had autonomic neuropathy.

Many doctors and cardiologists claim, "One aspirin a day will keep the heart attack away." However, aspirin is known for its antiplatelet ability. This means that it helps reduce or prevent clotting by decreasing platelet aggregation. In layman's terms, this keeps the blood thin. However, this comes at a cost—a pretty steep one, at that. Aspirin depletes the body of life-saving nutrients. These nutrients include folic acid, iron, potassium, sodium, and vitamin C. Depletion of these nutrients and minerals is directly correlated with the development or progression of polyneuropathy, as you will see in later chapters. Symptoms associated with such depletion include elevated homocysteine, which is a risk factor for heart disease. (Oops! What happened to decreasing the risk for heart attacks?) These symptoms also include headaches, depression, and suppression of the immune system, to name just a few. Internal bleeding is also a real and present danger when taking aspirin, which always results in anemia.

There are much better clinically proven natural alternatives that will give you this same platelet protection without the risks and side effects. One such natural alternative is taking vitamin E on a daily basis. Vitamin E not only helps prevent thick, sticky blood—a problem in cardiovascular disease—it also offers significant protection against neuropathy and nerve damage.

The side effects of aspirin are so severe that they can result in death. Each year, a grossly underestimated 7,600 deaths and 76,000 hospitalizations occur in the United States from use of aspirin and other NSAIDS, such as Motrin, Aleve, and Celebrex. The CDC estimates that only 10 percent of deaths caused by NSAIDS are reported.

Much to my dismay, these drugs are not the only culprits involved in creating peripheral neuropathy. There are many other prescription medications that can cause peripheral nerve damage and create polyneuropathy as a side effect. Even several of the well-known drugs used to treat neuropathic pain create more nerve damage, as a side effect. This sounds outlandish, but unfortunately, it's very true. I've enclosed a list for you.

Neuropathy is typically brought about by the damage caused by the toxic effects of drugs on peripheral nerves. Damage commonly occurs at the axon of the nerves.

A study of medication-induced neuropathies published by Dr. Louis H. Weimer, MD, found that "Numerous medications have been associated with neuropathy, but many more agents (medications) are suspected of causing neurotoxicity, including peripheral neuropathy, than have convincing proof. Also, many subclinical or unsuspected cases likely remain undiagnosed." He further concludes in his research article that "Medication-induced toxicity should be at least considered in new cases of neuropathy including apparent idiopathic forms. Also important, patients with existing neuropathy of known or presumed cause should have their current regimen and planned therapy considered for neurotoxicity." (7)

www.neuropathydoctorsa.com

MEDICATIONS KNOWN TO CAUSE NEUROPATHY

The following is a list of medications that have been shown to cause neuropathy as a side effect

Anticonvulsants / Neuropathy
Gabapentin (Neurontin)
Pregabalin
Lyrica
Phenytoin (Dilantin®)
Duloxetine hydrochloride

Peripheral Neuropathy
Allopurinol (Zyloprim)
Amiodarone (Cordarone)
Amitriptyline (Elavil)
Lotrel
Metrogl (Metrogel)

Antibiotics:
Cipro
Flagyl
Levaquin (Levofloxacin)
Metronidazole

Anti-Alcohol Drug
Disulfiram

Antianxiety:
Ambien (Zolpidem)
BuSpar
Cymbalta
Klonopin (Clonazepam)
Xanax

Antidepressant:
Citalopram (Celexa)
Duloxetine (Cymbalta)
Venlafaxine (Effexor)
Effexor XR
Nortriptyline
Zoloft

Blood Pressure or Heart Medications:
Amiodarone/Cordarone
Atenolol
Aceon
Ramipril (Altace)
Cozaar
Hydralazine
Hydrochlorothiazide (HCT)
Hydrodiuril
Hyzaar
Lisinopril
Micardis
Norvasc
Prazosin
Prinivil
Ramipril
Zestril

Chemotherapy Drugs
Cisplatin
Vincristine (Oncovin)
Carboplatin (Paraplatin)
Paclitaxel (Taxol),
Nab-Paclitaxel (Abraxane)
Docetaxel (Taxotere)
Ixabepilone (Ixempra)
Vinblastine (Velban, Alkaban-Aq),
Vincasar Pes, (Vincrex),
Vinorelbine (Navelbine),
Etoposide (Toposar, Vepesid, Etopophos)
Thalidomide (Thalomid)
Lenalidomide (Revlimid)
Bortezomib (Velcade)
Eribulin Mesylate (Halaven)
Herceptin

Cholesterol Lowering Drugs:
Advicor
Altocor
Atorvastatin
Baycol (removed from market d/t death)
Caduet
Cerivastatin
Crestor
Fluvastatin
Lescol
Lescol XL
Lipex
Lipitor
Lipobay
Lopid
Lovastatin
Mevacor
Pravachol
Pravastatin
Pravigard Pac
Rosuvastatin
Simvastatin
Vytorin
Zocor

Dental Creams:
all zinc containing creams including:
Polygrip
Fixodent

HIV Drugs:
d4T (Zerit)
ddC (Hivid)
ddI (Videx EC)

5

WHAT YOUR DOCTOR DIDN'T TELL YOU!

"A healthy body is a guest-chamber for the soul; a sick body is a prison."

Virgil
(70–19 BC)

Causes of Neuropathy

There are many causes of neuropathy. We saw in the previous chapter the correlation between medications and peripheral nerve damage. Chronic neuropathy can begin when your nerves undergo a state of anoxia. This is a condition in which the nerve is deprived of oxygen. Nerves can also become damaged when they are poisoned by continual exposure to toxic chemicals, which accumulate in the body. There are a variety of reasons why this might happen. Quite commonly, we see a combination of reasons.

Some of the most common causes are:

- Diabetes
- Medications
- Chemotherapy/Radiation
- Surgeries or other physical injuries
- Heavy Metals (lead, mercury, chromium, arsenic, etc.)
- Environmental chemicals and toxins (MSG, aspartame, pesticides, etc.)
- Malnutrition / nutritional deficiencies caused by:
    a) lack of nutrients in food and/or processed food
    b) inability of digestive tract to absorb nutrients eaten due to acid reflux, gluten intolerance, food sensitivities, Crohn's disease, diverticulitis, colitis, IBS, or other digestive disorders.

Let's take a look at how some of these conditions can create peripheral neuropathies. When we examine the statistic of the twenty-two million people who are affected yearly by polyneuropathy, surprisingly, only seven million cases are caused by diabetes. The remaining fifteen million are non-diabetes related. When I first learned of this statistic, it blew my mind. As doctors, one of the first things we learn is that diabetes and neuropathy go hand in hand. To discover that there are actually more cases of people suffering from neuropathy who don't have diabetes—that was shocking.

Diabetes and Neuropathy

Our long-standing war on diabetes in the United States is turning into more of a massacre. Diabetes is responsible for a vast number of secondary illnesses and disorders. Diabetic patients struggle to control their levels of glucose (or blood sugar) on a daily basis. As a result, they suffer from high levels of glucose in their blood over an extended period of time, which carries enormous consequences. When we look at the number of people afflicted with diabetes, we find that 60 to 70 percent of all diabetics will develop polyneuropathy. Researchers have long been studying how prolonged exposure to high blood glucose causes nerve damage.

With regard to neuropathies, chronically elevated glucose levels can damage blood vessels that carry oxygen and nutrients to the nerves. This can lead to anoxia—a lack of oxygen to the nerve cells and blood vessels—which can result in poor circulation and nerve damage. This is a large part of the reason that most neuropathy sufferers have not only pain but also abnormal changes in the skin on the legs. These changes can include purple discolorations, extremely dry, flaky skin, and extremely taut skin. All of these things are signs that the skin has lost proper circulation and thus oxygenation and nutrients; it also signifies that the skin is beginning to die.

New evidence correlates metabolic syndrome with small fiber damage leading to neuropathy.

Metabolic syndrome, also known as metabolic syndrome X, is the name applied to a group of risk factors that raises your risk for cardiovascular disease, stroke, and diabetes. It is becoming more prevalent in the United States with each passing year. Researchers have found that one thing is for certain:

all of the risk factors associated with metabolic syndrome are related to obesity.

The six conditions described below (taken from the *American Heart Association*'s guidelines and NIDH) are metabolic risk factors. You must have at least three metabolic risk factors to be diagnosed with metabolic syndrome.

- Elevated waist circumference *(apple-shaped body)*:
    Men—greater than 40 inches (102 cm)
    Women—greater than 35 inches (88 cm)
- Elevated triglycerides: Equal to or greater than 150 mg/dL ('mg' stands for milligrams and dL stands for deciliter. This is a standard unit of measure in blood work that shows the concentration of a substance—like triglycerides—in a specific amount of fluid, such as blood)

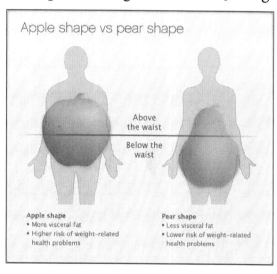

- Reduced HDL ("good") cholesterol:
    Men—less than 40 mg/dL
    Women—less than 50 mg/dL
- Elevated blood pressure: Equal to or greater than 130/85 mm Hg, or use of medication for hypertension
- Elevated fasting glucose: Equal to or greater than 100 mg/dL, or use of medication for hyperglycemia

- Insulin resistance: Hemoglobin A1C levels equal to or greater than 6.0

The tests that may be done to diagnose metabolic syndrome include:

- Blood pressure measurement
- Glucose test
- Hemoglobin A1c (HbA1c)
- HDL cholesterol level
- LDL cholesterol level
- Total cholesterol level
- Triglyceride level

1. **The two most important risk factors for metabolic syndrome:** Extra weight around the middle and upper parts of the body, also known as central obesity.
2. Insulin resistance.

What is Insulin Resistance?

Insulin, a hormone made by the pancreas, helps the body get glucose into the cells. Glucose, a form of sugar, is the main energy source or fuel for the cells of your body. It is much like gasoline is to your car. During the process of digestion, food is broken down into glucose, which then travels in the bloodstream to cells throughout the body. When glucose is circulating in the bloodstream it is called blood glucose, also known as blood sugar. After a meal, your blood glucose level rises, signaling the pancreas to release insulin.

One of the actions of insulin is to cause the cells of the body, particularly the muscle and fat cells, to remove glucose from the blood by opening up a door or channel into the cell. Insulin has the ability to do this by binding to a specific receptor on the surface of the cell. Think of this receptor site as a lock on a door, and think of insulin as the key that unlocks this door, allowing it to open. Insulin (the key) slides into the lock (receptor site on a cell). If the lock is not damaged, the key should open the door to the cell, so that glucose gets in. If the lock, (the cell receptor site) is damaged, the key may fit in, but it will not turn and unlock the door. If this happens, glucose can't get into the cell, where it can be used as energy. This leaves high levels of glucose circulating in the blood. We call this **insulin resistance.** With increased levels of glucose in the blood, the pancreas is signaled to produce more insulin in the hope that additional "keys" might open the cell door. Once the cell is resistant to insulin, this will set off an alarm in the pancreas, causing it to continuously produce increased levels of insulin. Eventually, the pancreas will be unable to keep up with the body's demands for more insulin, and it will fail. This will cause excess glucose to build up in the bloodstream, setting the stage for type 2 diabetes. If a person becomes insulin resistant and does not take the necessary steps to reverse it (and yes, it can be reversed!), they will end up with diabetes. It's not a matter

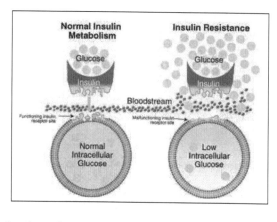

of *if* they develop diabetes but more a matter of *when* they will develop diabetes.

A study published in the *New England Journal of Medicine* in 2005 revealed the correlation between small fiber neuropathy and metabolic syndrome. One study involving 548 patients with type 2 diabetes showed that those with metabolic syndrome were twice as likely to have neuropathy as those without the syndrome.

Research findings strongly suggest that even prediabetes is a risk factor for small fiber neuropathy. Nerves do not require insulin for glucose uptake. Therefore, diabetics accumulate excess glucose in their nerves. Glucose in nerve cells can cause free radical damage. It also causes a large decrease in multiple nutrients and antioxidants, such as vitamin C, taurine, carnitine, and inositol. All of these nutrients are necessary for nerve conduction and transmission. Elevated glucose levels also lead to a decreased production in nitric oxide (NO). A lack of NO production oftentimes leads to vascular impairment, which means damage to blood vessels. This will take you down a path that will lead directly to neuropathy's door.

It is equally important to realize that glucose levels in the blood can spike to nerve-damaging levels after a meal, even if your fasting and average blood glucose levels remain below normal levels. Normal levels are currently considered to be below one hundred for fasting blood plasma and below 6.0 for HGBA1c (hemoglobin A1c, the test commonly used to measure insulin sensitivity). Studies have shown that many of the cases of small fiber peripheral neuropathy with symptoms of tingling, pain, and loss of sensation in the feet and hands are due to a glucose intolerance found before a diagnosis of diabetes or prediabetes has ever been reached. This damage is much easier to reverse with diet, exercise, and weight loss, particularly because it occurs in the very early stages of neuropathy.

Chemotherapy-Induced Peripheral Neuropathy (CIPN)

Chemotherapy drugs are poisons that attack rapidly dividing cells (fast-growing cells). These drugs do not differentiate between healthy and diseased cells when they attack, thereby destroying healthy cells along with the mutated cells. The theory behind using these toxins is that they will destroy the fast-growing cancer cells before doing too much damage to normal cells.

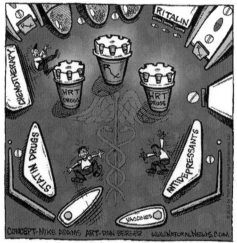

Unfortunately, chemotherapy is hardest on the nervous system. Nerve cells are more sensitive than most other cells to these toxins. It is reported that neuropathy is a common and expected part of treatment with the following chemotherapy drugs: platins (cisplatin, oxaliplatin), vincristine, taxols (paclitaxel and docetaxel), and more recently, with bortezomib. After one has been exposed to chemotherapy, damage can occur to the myelin producing cells (fatty sheath that helps insulate and protect nerve). Chemotherapy causes nerve damage, paving the way for a common side effect, peripheral neuropathy.

Patients taking cisplatin often experience peripheral neuropathy as a side effect. The symptoms they describe are numbness and tingling. On examination, they show a loss of deep-tendon reflexes. Cisplatin has a direct impact on the calcium channel's ability to function properly to generate a nerve impulse. German scientists have studied the channel currents based on calcium, sodium, and phosphorus, and the effect of the addition of cisplatin.

Their studies revealed that cisplatin directly affects calcium balance. They also discovered that the addition of cisplatin reduced the normal activity of the calcium channels. The theory is that cisplatin enters the neuron and slows the response of the calcium channels. Cisplatin typically affected the small neurons, making this finding consistent with the patients' symptoms. Small neurons are responsible for sensory responses, whereas large neurons play more of a role in motor processes.

Nervous system damage might not always manifest immediately in chemotherapy patients. The onset of these symptoms is variable. Certain drugs might cause symptoms during or immediately after the first dose in some patients, while others might experience a delayed onset of symptoms up to several weeks, months, or even years after their last dose. The severity of the neuropathy symptoms will be proportionate to the cumulative dosage of the drug received. Regardless of the cause, someone with preexisting neuropathy might develop a more severe and longer-lasting neuropathy.

Signs and symptoms of CIPN include sensory impairment (damage to nerves that transmit sensations of light touch, vibration, position, temperature, and pain perception), motor impairment (damage to nerves controlling muscles under conscious control—walking, grasping objects, buttoning a shirt, etc.), and autonomic impairments (damage to nerves controlling organs under involuntary control—heart, bladder, colon, etc.). Other common signs of CIPN are loss of deep-tendon reflexes or sensory deficits such as numbness and tingling in the hands and feet, also referred to as stocking-glove distribution. Motor impairments with CIPN can include symmetrical muscle weakness. It can also include a severe condition known as foot or wrist drop. Foot drop is the inability to point the toes or ankle upward. Foot drop may include muscle weakness of the forefoot, making it difficult to raise the foot up when walking, or it could be as severe as complete paralysis of the foot. Wrist drop is a condition in which damage to the radial nerve of the wrist prevents the person from extending the wrist, causing it to hang limply.

Oxaliplatin can cause both acute and chronic neuropathy. The acute process can begin within minutes of injecting the drug into the vein and it can cause immediate numbness, tingling or burning of the hands, feet, throat, and mouth area; the chronic form is a dose-dependent sensory neuropathy that is similar to other chemotherapy-induced neuropathies. Vincristine can cause sore throats and constipation, along with other motor neuropathic deficits.

Surgeries / Physical Injuries and Neuropathy

Physical injuries or any form of trauma—such as car accidents, falls, or sport injuries—can cause injury to a nerve by creating a stretch, compression, or crushing injury. Nerves can also be severed or forcibly detached from the spinal cord, either partially or completely. Less severe traumas, such as fractured or dislocated bones, can cause serious nerve damage by exerting pressure on neighboring nerves. Disc herniation, protrusion, and bulges between vertebrae can compress nerve fibers where they emerge from the spinal cord, thereby damaging the nerve and creating neuropathic pain. These are only a few types of injuries that might induce neuropathy.

Oftentimes, we do not think of surgery as a bodily trauma or injury, but it is. Any time the tissues of your body are disrupted, whether intentionally or accidentally, the body processes the mechanism as an assault on the tissue. As such, the body will go through the same cascade of healing. It's not uncommon for neuropathy to develop as a side effect of surgery. During the course of surgery, nerves might be damaged, either directly (i.e., the nerve is severed or nicked) or indirectly (i.e., the nerve is bruised or the tissue surrounding the nerve is inflamed, leading to nerve compression). For example, the way in which a patient is positioned during a surgical procedure can indirectly cause neuropathy. Maintaining a patient in a prolonged position can hamper circulation and deprive the nerve of oxygen and necessary nutrients. These prolonged periods of positioning can also create an abnormal stretch or compression on the nerve. Any of these situations can lead to nerve damage.

Symptoms of surgical nerve injury can include numbness and tingling or a burning pain, which can be moderate to severe. The symptoms might occur at the surgical site or in the standard areas where one typically observes peripheral neuropathy (i.e., feet, legs, hands, and arms). Sometimes, a person will notice that the symptoms worsen with specific motions or movements, or while he or she is sleeping at night.

Alcohol Abuse and Neuropathy

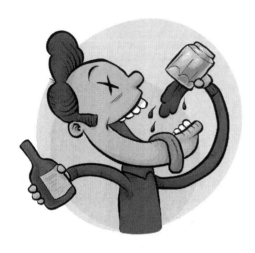

Alcoholic neuropathy, as it's called, is a neurological disorder in which multiple peripheral nerves throughout the body begin to malfunction simultaneously. This develops as a result of direct poisoning of the nerves by the alcohol. Degeneration of the nerves will typically occur in both the motor and sensory systems. This type of nerve damage will cause an individual to experience pain and muscular weakness. As is the case with most neuropathies, this will occur first in the feet and hands, and then it will progressively affect the central core. In alcoholic neuropathy, the main cause of damage to the nerves is the direct toxic effect that alcohol has on the nerve. However, vitamin deficiencies resulting from poor nutrition associated with alcoholism are also known to contribute to its development.

Long-term heavy alcohol use (dependence), or alcoholism, can inhibit or impair your body's ability to use and store certain vitamins and minerals. This will create a vitamin deficiency within the body, which in turn can lead to a polyneuropathy.

Prolonged and heavy alcohol consumption can lead to a loss of appetite, decreased food intake, and damage to the lining of the gastrointestinal (GI) tract. Inflammation and damage to the GI tract reduces the absorption of nutrients consumed. We refer to this state as malnutrition. Nerves are totally dependent on a continuous and reliable supply of both oxygen and glucose from the blood for normal, healthy functioning. In cases of prolonged or severe malnutrition, nerve function deteriorates as the body's energy reserves are depleted.

> 1. Thiamin (B1), Niacin (B3), Biotin (B7), and (B12) methyl cobalamin promote healthy nerves.
>
> 2. Riboflavin (B2) aids in nerve insulation.
>
> 3. Pyridoxine (B6) necessary for absorption of B3 and B12.
>
> 4. B6 and B7 reduce nerve pain.
>
> 5. B9 (folic acid) and B12 deficiency can cause neuropathic leg and foot pain.

It is important to recognize that neuropathies can develop with a significant depletion in any of the family of B vitamins and various other vitamins. Vitamins E, B1, B6, B12, and niacin are essential to healthy nerve function. Thiamine is a critical vitamin that is necessary for nourishment and the healthy functioning of the nervous system. Deficiencies in these vitamins can cause a painful neuropathy of the extremities. Aside from the roles they play in the peripheral nerves, both thiamine and niacinamide are required for normal brain functioning and cognitive activity, and they can aid in energy production. We will cover this in greater depth in the nutritional section.

Alcoholic polyneuropathy usually has a gradual onset, occurring over the course of many months or even years. Typically, axonal degeneration will begin before any symptoms arise. One early warning sign of the possibility of developing alcoholic polyneuropathy is weight loss. This usually signifies multiple nutritional deficiencies that lead to the development of polyneuropathy.

As is common in most neuropathies, symptoms will consist of both sensory and motor loss, and it will then develop symmetrically on both sides of the body. Individuals will ordinarily notice that it feels like they are wearing stockings or gloves.

Common symptoms of sensory involvement include numbness or abnormal sensations, such as feeling pins and needles in the legs or arms, and heat intolerance. Some people might notice a burning sensation in their feet and calves. Sensory symptoms will prevail first, only then to be followed by motor symptoms. These can include muscle cramps and weakness, muscle wasting, and decreased or absent deep tendon reflexes. Some people might experience frequent falls and unsteadiness in their gait due to a lack of muscular strength. Other motor symptoms include erectile dysfunction in men, problems urinating, constipation, and diarrhea. Over time, alcoholic polyneuropathy may also cause difficulty swallowing (dysphagia) and speech impairment.

Environmental Toxins and Neuropathy

Toxin accumulation within the body can cause peripheral nerve damage. What are toxins, and where do they come from? Toxins are chemicals that we absorb into our body. They come from the food that we eat (pesticides, phthalates, MSG, aspartame, etc.), plastic contain-

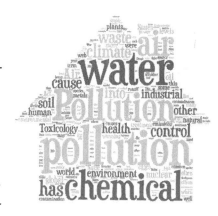

ers that food and beverages are packed in, the water that we drink (chlorine, fluoride, heavy metals), household cleaners, personal care products, makeup, and perfumes and colognes, to name a few.

Our bodies are designed to naturally detoxify unwanted substances daily, as part of normal metabolic functioning. Detoxification is one of the body's most basic automatic functions—eliminating and neutralizing toxins through the colon, liver, kidneys, lungs, skin, and lymphatic system. Unfortunately, in this day and age, with the pollution found in the air, water, and food, our bodies have an incredibly difficult time keeping up to the demands.

Nerve damage can occur when we are exposed to natural or artificial toxic substances. These toxins are called neurotoxins. Neurotoxins are destructive and poisonous to the nervous system, thereby altering the normal activity of the nerves. This can eventually disrupt and damage nerve cells.

TOP 10 LIST OF MOST COMMON TOXINS	
ENVIRONMENT	**HOUSHOLD**
1. Heavy Metals 2. PCB's 3. Dioxins 4. Pesticides 5. Phthalates and Plasticides 6. VOC's (volatile organic compounds) 7. Asbestos 8. Chlorine and Chloroform 9. Lead, Arsenic 10. Fluoride	1. Aluminum 2. PTFE and PFOAs (Teflon, Calphalon) 3. Chlorine bleach 4. Dry-cleaning chemicals 5. Household cleaners 6. Ammonia 7. Personal care products 8. Insecticides 9. BPA (Bisphenol-A) 10. Perfluorinated chemicals (carpet, upholstery stain protection)

People who are exposed to neurotoxins in the form of heavy metals (arsenic, lead, mercury, and thallium), industrial chemicals, or environmental toxins frequently develop neuropathy.

One of the most common heavy metals that people are exposed to is mercury. Mercury has been known to cause illness since the ancient Roman times, and it has been documented as neurotoxic, which means that it has the ability to poison and kill nerves. According to US government agencies, mercury and other heavy metals cause adverse health effects and learning disabilities in millions of people in the United States each year. The elderly and children are especially susceptible.

Mercury is by far one of the most pervasive heavy metals that we are dealing with in the twenty-first century. It can be found in our oceans, soil, water, air, and teeth. Mercury is a metal that has been used in products such as dental amalgams (silver fillings), light bulbs, batteries, paint, and thermometers. Due to the major pollution and toxic waste run-off occurring in our oceans, lakes, and streams, it is well known that many of our marine wildlife are carrying high concentrations of mercury within their bodies.

There are several forms of mercury:

1. <u>Elemental (metallic) mercury</u>: This refers to a shiny, silver, odorless liquid that is used in thermometers. It is absorbed by the body through vapors.

2. <u>Organic mercury</u>: This refers to mercury combined with carbon. The most common form is methyl mercury, which can be found in the fish that we consume. Another organic form of mercury is found in thimerosol, a preservative used in vaccines, including the influenza vaccine, and personal

care products like contact lens solutions. One study revealed that ingestion of thimerosol in adults led to multisystemic toxicities, including peripheral neuropathy. Mercury can be absorbed through the digestive tract and through vapors in the mouth and nasal passageways. Organic mercury is soluble in lipids (fats), and it can easily cross the blood-brain barrier and the placenta. Since your brain is the most important organ in your body—controlling all of your functions—your body created a specialized filtering mechanism called the blood-brain barrier (BBB). The BBB is a protective barrier that separates circulating blood and cerebrospinal fluid (CSF), the clear fluid that surrounds the spinal cord and brain and acts as a shock absorber. This barrier aids in selectively allowing necessary nutrients to pass into the brain while keeping out certain harmful substances, such as bacteria, viruses, drugs, and chemicals. To help paint a clearer picture, think of your BBB as a kitchen strainer. If you are draining spaghetti, you would place it in a strainer to let the water run through, while keeping the spaghetti in; however, if you rinse the spaghetti and it has chopped herbs on it, the herbs might still pass through the strainer. Mercury, like the dried herbs in this example, has the ability to pass through, or cross, the BBB.

3. <u>Inorganic mercury</u>: This refers to mercury combined with noncarbon substances. Mercury salts are one kind of inorganic mercury. This form of mercury has been used in medicines. Mercuric nitrate was used by the felt-hat industry in the process of curing felt. People in the felt-hat industry sometimes showed signs of mercury poisoning and came down with Mad Hatter syndrome. This is

where the phrase "mad as a hatter" originated, and it was the basis for the Mad Hatter character in one of my all-time favorite books, *Alice in Wonderland*. In 1941, the US finally banned the use of mercuric nitrate in the hat industry.

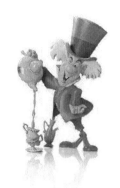

All three forms of mercury are toxic and destructive to the nervous system. Methyl mercury targets and kills neurons in specific areas of the nervous system, including the brain, making it especially dangerous to developing babies. This form of mercury is highly toxic, and it can cross the placenta and the blood-brain barrier. Mercury will then become concentrated in the brain of the developing fetus because the metal is absorbed quickly and is not excreted out of the body efficiently. Because of the damage that mercury incites in nerves, children exposed to mercury might be born with symptoms resembling cerebral palsy, spasticity, and other movement abnormalities, convulsions, visual problems, and abnormal reflexes.

Mercury amalgam dental fillings have been found to be the largest source of both inorganic and methyl mercury in people who have several amalgam fillings. Nearly 200 million people in the USA alone still have silver fillings.

> **Dental amalgams—silver fillings**
>
> 80 % of mercury vapors enter the body daily from mercury amalgams (silver fillings) causing mercury exposure in a person to be ten times greater than someone that does not have mercury amalgams.

These fillings continuously release mercury as a toxic vapor, and as much as 80 percent of the vapor enters the body. Until recently, people assumed that the mercury stayed within the filling. Now it is known that **mercury leaches out of the filling and into the mouth, digestive tract, and nasal passageways every minute of the day.** The average amalgam filling releases about thirty-four micrograms of mercury daily. Hundreds of thousands of medical lab tests identified mercury exposure levels to be ten times greater than the average level for people without amalgams. They also found that mercury excretion levels declined by 90 percent after the amalgam was replaced. If you would like to learn more about other diseases and illnesses linked with mercury toxicity, I highly recommend reading *The Poison in Your Teeth* by Dr. Tom McGuire, DDS. Also, visit http://iaomt.org/videos/ to watch the video titled, "The Smoking Teeth." It's an extremely interesting eight-minute video that demonstrates the mercury vapor being released from a tooth and the effects that this has on the nervous system and other organ systems in the body. I often play this video when I give public lectures. You will likely find it very enlightening.

It's important for us to discuss the role that fish consumption can play in adding mercury into your body. Fish and shellfish have many nutritional benefits. Fish and shellfish contain high-quality protein and other essential nutrients. They are low in saturated fat, and they contain omega-3 fatty acids. However, nearly all fish and shellfish contain trace amounts of methyl mercury. How does this element get into our fish supply? Mercury contamination can occur naturally, but it usually occurs in greater abundance from man-made sources. Some of it can be traced to coal-burning power plants; smokestacks release toxic mercury emissions,

> Mercury damages and kills nerves in both the central nervous system and peripheral nervous system.

which rain down into rivers, lakes, and oceans. Bacteria convert the mercury to a form that's easily absorbed by insects and other small organisms. Mercury moves up the food chain as small fish eat the small organisms and big fish eat the smaller fish. The highest concentrations accumulate in large predators such as sharks, swordfish, and tuna—some of America's favorite fish. Certain types of fish and shellfish contain higher levels of mercury, which can harm an unborn baby or young child's developing nervous system. The risks from mercury in fish and shellfish depend on the amounts eaten and the levels of mercury in the fish or shellfish. Remember, mercury has a cumulative effect within the body. The FDA issued a consumer advisory for women who might become pregnant or are currently pregnant, nursing mothers, and young children, warning them to avoid types of fish that contain higher levels of mercury and encouraging them to eat fish and shellfish that are lower in mercury.

This list has been formulated by the NRDC (National Resources Defense Council), and I have listed it here for you. You can also go to *www.nrdc.org* to see their full report and download a wallet-sized card to carry with you.

Protecting Yourself—and the Fish

Certain fish, even some that are low in mercury, are poor food choices for other reasons. Most often, they have been fished so extensively that their numbers are perilously low. These fish are marked with an asterisk.

FISH CONTAINING THE LEAST AMOUNT OF MERCURY

Anchovies
Butterfish
Catfish
Clam
Crab (Domestic)
Crawfish/Crayfish
Croaker (Atlantic)
Flounder*
Haddock (Atlantic)*
Hake
Herring
Mackerel (North Atlantic, Chub)
Mullet
Oyster
Perch (Ocean)
Plaice
Pollock
Salmon (Canned)*
Salmon (Fresh)*
Sardine
Scallop*

Shad (American)
Shrimp*
Sole (Pacific)
Squid (Calamari)
Tilapia
Trout (Freshwater)
Whitefish
Whiting

FISH CONTAINING A MODERATE AMOUNT OF MERCURY

Eat six servings or fewer per month:
Bass (Striped, Black)
Carp
Cod (Alaskan)*
Croaker (White Pacific)
Halibut (Atlantic)*
Halibut (Pacific)
Jacksmelt

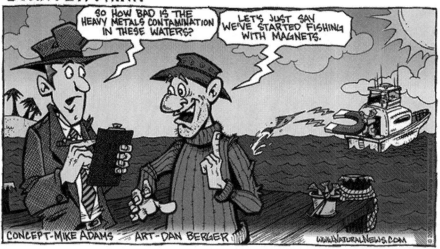

(Silverside)
Lobster
Mahi Mahi
Monkfish*
Perch (Freshwater)
Sablefish
Skate*
Snapper*
Tuna (Canned chunk light)
Tuna (Skipjack)*
Weakfish (Sea Trout)

FISH THAT ARE HIGH IN MERCURY

Eat three servings or fewer per month:
Bluefish
Grouper*
Mackerel (Spanish, Gulf)
Sea Bass (Chilean)*
Tuna (Canned Albacore)
Tuna (Yellowfin)*

FISH WITH THE HIGHEST LEVELS OF MERCURY

Avoid eating:
Mackerel (King)
Marlin*
Orange Roughy*
Shark*
Swordfish*

Tilefish*
Tuna (Bigeye, Ahi)*

Sources for NRDC's guide: The data for this guide to mercury in fish comes from two federal agencies: the Food and Drug Administration, which tests fish for mercury, and the Environmental Protection Agency, which determines mercury levels that it considers safe for women of childbearing age.

About the mercury-level categories: The categories on the list are determined according to the following mercury levels in the flesh of tested fish:

- Least mercury: <0.09 parts per million,
- Moderate mercury: 0.09–0.29 parts per million,
- High mercury: 0.3–0.49 parts per million,
- Highest mercury: > 0.5 parts per million.

The question racing through your brain at this point (if you haven't consumed too much fish, of course) is: "How exactly does mercury do all this damage?" Mercury is fat-soluble and it can enter every cell of your body through its lipid membranes. Cell membranes consist of approximately 60 percent protein and 40 percent fat. Nerve cells are an exception, containing nearly 75 percent fat. These fat-rich membranes determine what enters the cell and what does not. Methyl mercury oxidizes within the body into an extremely destructive form of mercury. Methyl mercury (the type of mercury found in silver fillings) is considered to be the most dangerous form, due to its ability to travel great distances and enter all cells in the body. Once inside the cell, mercury can disrupt the internal structures and metabolic pathways of the cell and kill off the neurons, both directly and indirectly.

Studies have found that mercury can kill or damage brain and nerve cells. Mercury can inhibit the production of neurotransmitters in the nerve by inhibiting normal calcium-channel function, as well as nitric oxide synthase. Nitric oxide is important for the function of nerve transmission.

Even at very low levels, mercury can inhibit nerve growth factors. Deficiencies in nerve growth factors result in nerve degeneration. A study conducted at the University of Calgary (Ontario) Medical School reported that mercury ions disrupt the membranes of young growing nerves, causing them to die back. This can severely inhibit and retard nerve regeneration. Mercury vapor, which is frequently released into the mouth with just one silver filling, is fat soluble. As you will recall, the myelin sheath of the nerve is made up of fat. As a result, mercury can easily deposit within the myelin sheath of the nerve, damaging the sheath and the nerve itself. Mercury also has an affinity for red blood cells and cells of the central nervous system. It only takes a few micrograms of mercury to severely disturb cellular function and inhibit nerve growth. There has been a huge increase in the incidence of degenerative neurological conditions in virtually all Western countries over the last two decades.

Although mercury toxicity may destructively target nerve tissues, it has an equally high affinity for the kidney. Mercury will not discriminate against kidney cell damage. After attacking these two areas, it can then wreak havoc in any tissue that might get in its way.

Certain dyes used in diagnostic studies like MRIs, CT scans, angiograms, and barium studies also have been linked with peripheral nerve damage. As a matter of fact, one of my patients stated that shortly after he received a dye for an angiogram study, he developed polyneuropathy, which affected his entire torso, legs, feet, arms, hands, and chest. He suffered with this polyneuropathy, which progressively worsened, for one year, until he began treatment at our clinic.

Chemicals in food

Another source of our toxic exposure comes from the highly processed and chemical-laden diets that we follow. Our American diet is loaded with too much animal protein, which contains hormones and antibiotics, too much trans-fat, too much caffeine, too many flavor enhancers, and too much alcohol. All of this radically overloads our natural detoxification pathways.

It is imperative for you to be aware that foods, especially processed foods, have additives that can cause nerve damage. Excitotoxins are so pervasive in our food supply that it's important that I touch on this topic. An excitotoxin is a chemical that causes brain cells and cells in the peripheral nervous system to become overexcited and fire uncontrollably. Ultimately, this will lead to the death of the cell. Excitotoxins are typically used as flavor enhancers in food or as artificial sweeteners in foods and beverages. The most common excitotoxins that we hear about are monosodium glutamate (MSG) and aspartame (Equal, NutraSweet). These substances have the potential to inflict permanent damage to the brain and the nervous system. These chemicals cross not only the blood-brain barrier but also the placental barrier, harming the brain and nervous system development of unborn children.

So, why are these harmful chemicals added to our foods? They enhance the flavor of food to the point of actually over-exaggerating. What do I mean by this? Excitotoxins have the ability to hyperstimulate our taste buds. Your tongue has special receptors for glutamate molecules, aka glutamic acid, which is an amino acid. Amino acids are the building blocks of proteins. This means that having a taste for glutamic acid is akin to having a taste for proteins, which are most commonly found in meat. Just as your sugar receptors give you a sweet tooth, your glutamate receptors give you a craving for meat and meaty flavors.

> **Patient—Rhonda**
>
> I was thirty-nine years old when I began experiencing severe pain, numbness, and tingling in my feet. I was diagnosed with neuropathy. It was so bad that it limited all of my activities. I began researching neuropathy and I discovered that diet could be a factor. At the time, I was drinking a lot of diet soda, which was sweetened with aspartame, every day. I learned that nerve damage is linked to aspartame, so I quit drinking all sodas and eliminated anything sweetened with aspartame. After doing this, my condition completely cleared up. I was amazed that a soft drink could create this amount of nerve damage. I will never touch another soda again!

MSG is a form of glutamate. When you add it to food, your food tastes meatier. Adding MSG to any dish makes it taste better. MSG is used in almost all processed foods, fast foods, and vegetarian meat substitute foods like veggie burgers, seitan, tofu dogs, tempeh bacon, etc.

Over the past several years MSG has become quite the hot topic. Consumers are becoming better acquainted with the dangers and risks of consuming MSG, and they are demanding that it be taken out of food. As a result, although the corporate food processors continue to add MSG to our foods, they are going to great lengths to disguise these harmful additives. For example, they use such deceptive names as vegetable protein, hydrolyzed vegetable protein, hydrolyzed plant protein, caseinate, yeast extract, and natural flavoring. When you see the phrase "natural flavors" on a food label, it is not a good thing, as you might think. If the flavoring were so natural, why wouldn't they simply list it on the label? Research has indicated that when these excitotoxin taste enhancers are combined, they become much more toxic than when they are alone.

READ THE LABEL

It's imperative to read the ingredients list on food labels. There are certain words that will indicate if a product contains MSG. I have compiled a list of ingredients that *always* contain MSG!

Terms Always Indicating Hidden MSG Additives

Autolyzed plant protein
Autolyzed yeast
Calcium caseinate
Gelatin
Glutamate Textured protein
Glutamic acid
Hydrolyzed Plant Protein (HPP)
Hydrolyzed protein

Hydrolyzed Vegetable Protein (HVP)
Monopotassium glutamate
Monosodium glutamate
MSG
Natural flavors
Sodium caseinate
Spices
Textured protein
Yeast extract
Yeast food
Yeast food nutrient

Terms Frequently Indicating Hidden MSG Additives

Malt extract
Bouillon
Broth
Stock
Flavoring
Natural Flavoring
Natural Beef or Chicken Flavoring
Seasoning
Spices

Additives that Sometimes Contain MSG or Excitotoxins

Carrageenan
Enzymes
Soy protein concentrate
Soy protein isolate
Whey protein concentrate

Body systems and organs that were once capable of cleaning out unwanted substances are now overloaded to the point that toxic material remains inside our tissues. These toxic substances will accumulate throughout the years, leading to possible neuropathies.

> *And we have made of ourselves living cesspools, and driven doctors to invent names for our diseases.*
>
> Plato
> (427–347 BC)

Systemic Illness and Neuropathy

There are many more causes of peripheral/polyneuropathy. I've devoted much of this book to highlighting the most common causes; however, I do want you to be aware of a list of other systemic chronic illnesses and disorders that can cause neuropathic pain.

Metabolic and Endocrine disorders

Nerve tissues are highly vulnerable to damage from diseases that impair the body's ability to transform nutrients into energy, process waste products, or manufacture the substances that make up living tissue. Diabetes is the most common and destructive of the metabolic disorders. We went into great detail about diabetes in previous chapters, but it's imperative to realize that any metabolic disorder that leads to impaired kidney function or kidney disease will also cause neuropathy. *Kidney disorders* can lead to abnormally high amounts of toxic substances in the blood, which can severely damage nerve tissue. A majority of patients who require dialysis because of kidney failure develop polyneuropathy. Some liver diseases, adrenal disorders, and thyroid dysfunctions have also been linked to the development of neuropathies as a result of chemical imbalances.

Infections and autoimmune disorders

Although less common, there are viruses and bacteria that are known to attack nerve tissues and cause peripheral neuropathy. I will briefly cover a few of these so that you will be familiar with them, but we will not spend a significant amount of time on the topic, since these conditions are less likely to occur.

1. Herpes varicella-zoster (shingles), Epstein-Barr virus, cytomegalovirus, and herpes simplex-members. These viruses severely damage sensory nerves, causing attacks of sharp, lightning-like pain. HIV, which causes AIDS, also creates extensive damage to the central and peripheral nervous systems. The best way to manage neuropathy caused by these viral infections is by decreasing systemic inflammation. I will share with you information on how you can achieve this in the chapter on nutrients and neuropathy. An important component, though, is detoxing your body and eliminating all processed foods. Switching to a healthy balanced diet is imperative when attempting to decrease inflammation throughout the body.

2. Bacterial infections such as Lyme disease are transmitted to humans through a bite by an infected tick. Lyme dis-

ease causes inflammation throughout the body, including the skin, the joints, and the nerves, which can cause extensive damage to the peripheral nerves. This infection can cause a wide range of neuropathic disorders, including a rapidly developing, painful polyneuropathy, often within a few weeks after initial infection by a tick bite.

3. Acute inflammatory demyelinating neuropathy, better known as Guillain-Barré syndrome, can damage motor, sensory, and autonomic nerve fibers. Guillain-Barre syndrome is a rare autoimmune disease that causes the cells of the immune system to attack the nerve cells. This causes damage to the nerves, which leads to tingling in the hands or feet and later can spread to the arms and legs. If not treated, the neuropathy can result in paralysis. The exact cause of Guillian-Barre syndrome is not known. However, the doctors at the Mayo Clinic report that 60 percent of cases are preceded by an infection.

4. Celiac disease is an autoimmune disease that is caused by sensitivity to gluten. Gluten is a protein found in highest concentration in wheat, barley and rye (gluten is found to a lesser degree in spelt, kamut, durum, semolina, bulgar and oats). When people who are sensitive to gluten eat foods that contain this protein, the immune system attacks the projections of the small intestine, called villi. These villi are responsible for the absorption of nutrients. When the villi become damaged, the body is unable to absorb and process the nutrients that you eat, resulting in malnutrition. The amount and quality

of the food that is consumed is irrelevant. Celiac disease is on the rise, affecting two million Americans.

5. The University of Chicago reports that approximately 10 percent of those with celiac disease suffer from peripheral neuropathy. It is imperative for people diagnosed with celiac disease to stay away from all sources of gluten and work toward healing the damage in their GI tract.

6. Certain autoimmune disorders will cause the destruction of the nerve's myelin sheath, such as multiple sclerosis, lupus, and rheumatoid arthritis. These autoimmune disorders also cause wide grade systemic inflammation and swelling, which will inadvertently damage nerve tissues. The key to minimizing neuropathy caused by autoimmune disorders is to decrease systemic inflammation, detoxify the body and eliminate all processed foods. Then adopt a healthy, balanced diet. This will aid in minimizing the damage to the nerves.

The above information will help give you a generalized overview of some of the other less common causes of neuropathy. It is important for anyone who may be afflicted by these disorders to realize that you might develop peripheral neuropathy as a result.

www.neuropathydoctorsa.com

6

PROVEN TREATMENTS TO REVERSE NEUROPATHY

"The first wealth is health."

–Ralph Waldo Emerson
(1803–1882)

As you have now learned, peripheral neuropathy has many causes and presentations. The treatment of neuropathy is aimed first at eliminating or controlling the cause. Second, treatment aims to maintain muscle strength and physical function, and third, it aims to eliminate symptoms such as neuropathic pain.

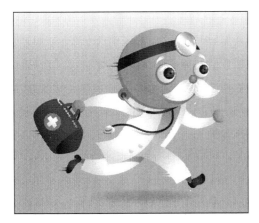

To get started with neuropathy care, proper treatment begins with proper diagnosis. Because of this, the first step to an accurate diagnosis is to perform a thorough medical history and physical examination. One would think that this is a no-brainer, right? After all, it is the standard of care. Unfortunately, in this day and age, when managed health care is always growing, nothing could be further from the truth. Due to stringent reductions in insurance reimbursements, rising medical equipment costs, and staff overhead, doctors are forced to increase their patient volume to make up for the lost revenue. As a result, it's common for you to walk into your doctor's office and wait for up to an hour or longer to be seen, merely to have the doctor spend ten minutes or less with you. These whopping ten minutes typically include the doctor reviewing your medical history and the examination. Oftentimes, many doctors even fail to perform an exam. There's nothing thorough about that.

When our patients come in for a consult and evaluation, we spend anywhere from twenty to thirty minutes of one-on-one time with them, gathering their medical history. I have found in my seventeen years of practice that there is no greater expert on a patient's body and its normal functioning than the patient themself. Unfortunately, most doctors no longer take the time to listen to their patients. They see this as a major inconvenience, slowing down the day's productivity. I can't begin to tell you how critical this first step is in evaluating a neuropathy patient's condition.

The next step, for our patients, involves a neurological examination. This is a very thorough exam, which includes quantitative sensory testing (QST) and skin vasomotor temperature testing. The latter test measures the inconsistencies in the distribution of skin temperature in any given area; it also assesses muscle strength, and it measures balance and proprioception. These tests are very accurate in diagnosing certain types of peripheral neuropathy, such as large and small fiber neuropathies, as seen with diabetes. The tests confirm the presence of neuropathy and they also assess the severity of the neuropathy. This is a necessary step in providing a baseline measurement, from which future progress can be assessed. QST testing is very useful in evaluating smaller caliber nerves by measuring pain and temperature thresholds to heat and cold. Large caliber nerves are evaluated by measuring thresholds of vibratory perception, joint position or proprioception, and sensory perception to touch stimuli.

In some cases, I might order electrodiagnostic studies, such as nerve conduction studies (NCS) and electromyelography (EMG), which are also very useful; however, these tests will not help with the diagnosis of small fiber neuropathy. Typically, by the time patients have walked through our doors, they have already had these tests performed. Quantitative sensory testing (QST) can be used to measure more objective changes in small fibers. Only after obtaining an extensive medical history and performing a detailed examination am I able to formulate a specific individualized treatment plan.

The traditional medical approach to treating neuropathy is to prescribe drugs to control the pain. This is not a treatment but merely a Band-Aid. At best, these drugs only mask or temper the pain. You have already seen earlier in this chapter that the very drugs that you are being prescribed can actually worsen your neuropathy. Most medical doctors, in fact, will tell you that there's no solution for healing or reversing your neuropathy. They will state, "You need to learn how to live with it." Well, this doesn't need to be the case. A research study done by the University of California, San Francisco (UCSF 2005, December) found that nerve regeneration is possible in spinal cord injuries. Another study by the American Academy of Neurology (AAN) revealed that "exercise and diet can reduce neuropathic pain and help regenerate nerve fibers in patients with impaired glucose tolerance (prediabetes)." There are many more studies that show that nerve regeneration is indeed possible. We regularly provide these to our patients. Quite often, their medical doctors have told them that their neuropathy is permanent and that nerve damage is irreversible. Many patients have bought into this inaccurate and downright false information. Part of our duty as their doctor is to reeducate them and show them the science behind nerve regeneration. I also encourage those who are bold enough to respectfully bring the studies to their doctors—or mail them—so that perhaps their doctors will become educated on the current research as well. If you would like to look at these research articles in further detail, visit my website: *www.neuropathydoctorsa.com*, where you

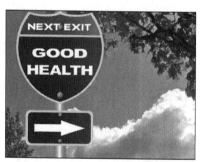

can download free copies.

You will hear me repeat this again and again: "The treatment for peripheral neuropathy depends on its cause." Therefore, the first step in treatment is to identify the cause.

- Vitamin deficiencies can be corrected.
- Diabetes can be controlled.
- Detoxifying the body can reverse neuropathies that are associated with toxic
- exposure.

- Nonsurgical techniques to remove the compression from the nerve can treat
- neuropathy that is caused by nerve entrapment.
- Nerves can regenerate under appropriate circumstances.

Because there are a vast number of causes of neuropathy, each person's treatment is customized based on their condition. As a result, it is imperative to treat neuropathy with a multifactorial approach. For instance, one patient came in to see us for his neuropathy, which had developed after having a diagnostic barium study performed. What I found was that this person's neuropathy, which had initially been brought on by toxicity from the barium, had worsened. The progression in his neuropathy was due to a continued assault on the nervous system from cholesterol medication and a diet laden with processed food chemicals. For this case, we first removed the initial offending agents by placing this patient on a whole system detoxification program. I then had to alter his dietary habits. As a result of this, when we ran new blood work, we found that the patient no longer suffered from elevated cholesterol, and therefore he no longer needed the cholesterol medication. Earlier, we discussed how statin drugs are an offending and precipitating agent for neuropathies. Next, I had to renourish the nerves so that his body had the necessary building blocks for repair.

On another case, I had a patient who suffered from uncontrolled diabetes, which was the cause of his neuropathy. This patient was taking gabapentin (Neurontin) in an attempt to control his neuropathy pain. I placed this patient on a low glycemic index diet and used nutritional support to aid his body with its ability to increase insulin sensitivity. The results for this patient were astounding. His pain was dramatically reduced, eliminating his need to take gabapentin. If you look back at the medication chart, you will see that gabapentin is yet another medication which can exacerbate or bring on neuropathy.

As you can see by the above examples, each case requires a customized approach to address all offending agents causing the neuropathy. Regardless of the initial cause of the neuropathy, there is always damage to the nerve tissue. To reverse this damage, all my patients receive our nonsurgical medical technology to stimulate, repair, and regenerate nerve tissue.

Since the causes of peripheral neuropathy can be very convoluted, I have developed a proprietary system of treatment using a combination of extremely advanced, drugless treatment procedures, which I call **Neurotrophic Restoration**™. These procedures include recently developed, noninvasive FDA-cleared medical equipment that utilizes Tesla technology. At our clinic, we do not utilize conventional EMS (electrical muscle stimulation) units, such as TENS, high-volt stimulation, low-volt galvanic stimulation, microcurrent, or interferential stimulation for neuropathy cases. This is the standard technology that is utilized by most medical clinics. Although this technology has a great degree of merit with regard to treating muscular injuries, it does not have the same level of efficacy in healing nerves. EMS units provide only superficial stimulation which merely eases surface muscle tension or spasm and masks the pain. You have already learned from reading this book that for a nerve to heal and regenerate, it takes a lot more than simply decreasing pain and easing muscle tension.

Our neurotrophic medical device, utilizing Tesla technology, allows for much deeper penetration of the stim-

ulation to the muscle fibers and blood vessels. What is truly remarkable about this technology is that it increases microcirculation of the blood vessels in the treated area by 300–500 percent. What this means for the neuropathy sufferer is that there is an increase in blood volume and blood flow, allowing for 300–500 percent greater oxygen delivery to the nerves, muscles, and blood vessels. This device also aids in the production of nitric oxide, which further improves circulation and increases nerve transmission. The Tesla technology also elicits deep fiber and lymphatic contraction, which enables edema (swelling), inflammation, and the associated toxins to be pumped out of the region. This results in decreased swelling, redness, and pain with increased nerve repair. It is truly amazing. I love watching the expressions on the patients' faces when they walk in with their feet and legs swollen and discolored in a purplish color and then leave after the treatment with their skin looking normal again. You cannot accomplish this deep degree of nerve repair and vascular improvement with a standard EMS machine. We then incorporate various other nonsurgical medical technology modalities to elicit the following: increased cellular energy and adenosine triphosphate (ATP), peripheral nerve stimulation, and restoring communication between the brain and the peripheral nervous system.

ATP is the energy fuel that is utilized by every cell within the body. It relates to your body like gasoline to your car. You might have a brand-new, shiny car but without gas in the tank, it is not going anywhere. In the case of nerve function, ATP is necessary for neurotransmitter production and nerve transmission. Every time a nerve fires, neurotransmitters must be replenished. ATP is responsible for the reformulation of your neurotransmitters. Any healing process within the body, including the peripheral nervous system, requires a great deal of ATP, so we use special technology that increases the production of ATP for the nerves. Our Neurotrophic Restoration™ system has common denominators of nerve repair, which are necessary components of healing, that are used on all patients, regardless of the cause of their neuropathy.

In addition, all of our patients receive neurotrophic nutrition to provide the building blocks for repair and regeneration of the nerves. This is a special formulation of nutrients, vitamins, and minerals, which I will go over in following chapters. They are important for nerve repair and regeneration. We have spent a significant amount of time researching the most effective combinations of nutrients to support nerve repair and regeneration as dictated by literature from medical journals and research. We have named this specialized formulation, Neuro-Gen™.

Whenever we devise a treatment protocol for our patients, we ensure that it always incorporates the following protocol:

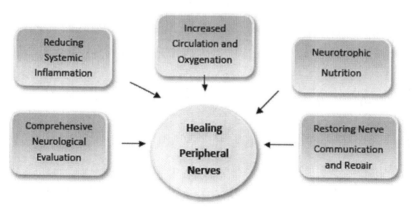

Another progressive and highly effective form of treatment that I use with my neuropathy cases is near infrared therapy. This is a precise form of noninvasive laser therapy with virtually no side effects, unlike medications prescribed for neuropathy. There are many different forms of infrared therapies on the market. However, not all will have the same efficacy on healing neuropathy; therefore, it's important to be familiar with the therapeutic benefits and differences of infrared.

To elicit healing in neuropathy cases, the infrared light wavelength must be in the range of 800 nm to 1,100 nm. This range will allow for penetration into tissues that are 10 cm–15 cm (4–6 inches) deep and it will trigger the release of nitric oxide (NO). Do not confuse nitric oxide (NO) with nitrous oxide, which is the laughing gas that some dental offices use as an anesthetic. NO is a molecule that is produced in the blood vessel wall by infrared light emitting diodes (LEDs) working within the frequencies of 800 nm and 1,100 nm. NO production stimulates cellular reproduction, relaxes muscles, promotes wound healing, stimulates collagen production, and most important, stimulates nerve transmission. NO is also beneficial for increasing circulation, which aids in delivering oxygen and nutrients to the nerves in the area, as well as in repairing damaged tissues. Last but not least, NO stimulates the production of endorphins. We like to call this the happy hormone because endorphins decrease pain signals. Beware, not all infrared devices operate at the same wavelength of light. Many infrared devices operate at wavelengths between 600 nm and 780 nm. At these wavelengths, the tissue penetration of light is not as deep, and it will not elicit the production of nitric oxide. Although a laser operating between 600 nm and 780 nm will have certain therapeutic benefits, it will be ineffective in repairing and regenerating nerves.

The final stage to healing the peripheral nerve is restoring proper communication pathways between the brain and the nerves of the feet or hands. This is imperative in order to return a person back to normal function. When your peripheral nerves become damaged, your brain will create new pathways to get the information to the impaired nerve. Unfortunately, the information may never reach its destination, or may be incomplete. This is a large contributing factor to balance problems which can lead to falls. In our treatment protocol, we restore the proper nervous system pathways by using a system called Quantum Sensory Techniques, which creates what we refer to as a Nervous System 'Reboot'. This approach lays down new and correct pathways of communication, allowing for the information from the brain to reach the appropriate destination. This enables improved balance and stability and reduces the incidence of falls.

In our modern world, in addition to the physical or chemical assault on your nervous system (leading to neuropathy), the average person is deficient in both vitamins and minerals. This is the main reason that I prescribe a formulation of supplements that are specific for the individual needs of my patients. This is a vital component to help repair and regenerate the damaged nerves.

> Near infrared lasers (NIR) must work within the frequency of 800–1100 nm to facilitate nerve repair and regeneration.

Early on in our practice, we would only utilize one modality at a time for a patient in an effort to keep costs low. What we discovered with this approach was that our results were very unpredictable and inconsistent. Through extensive research, we were able to formulate our multifactorial approach using various medical devices to accelerate the healing process of neuropathy. We would target nerve healing and regeneration from multiple directions, which has allowed us to achieve predictable results of an 80 percent patient satisfaction rate.

7

THE FOODS YOU EAT MAY BE KILLING YOUR NERVES

"The doctor of the future will give no medicine but will interest his or her patients in the care of the human frame, in a proper diet, and in the cause and prevention of disease."

Thomas Edison
(1847–1931)

As the obesity rate soars in the United States, Americans are more malnourished and mineral deficient than ever before. We live in a time when nutritional deficiency is unavoidable unless we are proactive. Our soil has become overcultivated to the point that it has been stripped of its rich mineral sources. This in turn makes the food grown in it mineral deficient. The food grown today does not have the same nutrient content or density that it had one hundred years ago. Our food is transported across the United States and internationally, increasing the storage time before it makes it to your table. This minimizes the vitality and nutrients of the foods that were once freshly picked. As if this were not bad enough, as the mainstay of our diet we now consume industrial by-products masquerading as food. You know what I'm talking about. Those processed sausage patties, fake butter, frozen food, and fast food. Yes, IHOP is a fast-food restaurant. Americans today eat out more often than ever before. We consume soft drinks by the gallon and water by the drops.

Large is the New Small

One of the biggest health issues in the US is obesity. It has reached epidemic proportions and the numbers are still escalating. It's no secret how this happened. As we have become more technologically advanced, our lives have become more sedentary and demands on our time have grown more stringent. People are exercising less than ever before in history. Families no longer sit down for a home-cooked, healthy meal. Meals are eaten on the run at popular places like McDonald's, Wendy's, KFC, Chick-fil-A, and Subway—and the list goes on. To get a better understanding of this, let's look at a few statistics from over the last one hundred years:

Obesity Statistics

36% of adults are obese.

30% of adults are overweight.

17% of youth are overweight or obese.

(Totaling 83% of the population battling weight issues-National Health and Nutrition Examination Survey, adults, children)

➢ Sugar consumption has increased from five pounds to 158 pounds per person per year.

➢ Chips, crackers, and other processed grains consumption has increased by sixty-two pounds per person per year.
➢ Soft drink consumption has increased by fifty-three gallons per person per year.
➢ Cheese consumption, including processed cheeses, has increased per person by twenty-eight pounds per year.
➢ The average American eats out between four and five times per week.
➢ Over the past seventy years, TV viewing has increased to 4.7 hours per day.

With this trend, it's no wonder that diabetes and metabolic syndrome are out of control. It also comes as no surprise that the people are being poisoned by toxic preservatives in all of the commercially prepared foods that they are consuming. As you will recall, these chemicals can cause peripheral neuropathy. Most processed and commercially prepared foods are loaded with toxins:

- Neurotoxic sweeteners
- Processed salt (devoid of natural trace minerals)
- Artificial flavors
- Trans fats
- Food colorings
- Preservatives and chemicals

The first thing you need to do is ensure that you are supplying your body with the right tools, allowing you to combat nutritional deficiency neuropathy. This means maintaining a healthy diet and a strong digestive process. Almost everyone's digestion today is very weak. This is caused by eating poor quality, refined, or processed foods, as well as having to digest so many chemicals in the food. **Weak digestion and poor eating habits impair the absorption of nutrients.** You don't have a digestive condition, you say. If you have fewer than two solid bowel movements per day, if you have bloating after meals, gas, or belching, if you suffer from indigestion (even occasionally), or worse, acid reflux—you have a digestive condition.

Modern Malnutrition

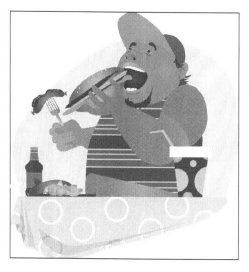

When we think of malnutrition, we typically think of third-world countries, where hunger and starvation run rampant—countries with poor water supplies and suboptimal living conditions. We picture poor emaciated children with stick-like arms and legs and bellies that are swollen and distended from a lack of food. We don't commonly think of America, the land of abundance, as being a country stricken with malnutrition, but it is. In fact, most obese people are malnourished. "How can this be?" you might ask, since this seems like an insane contradiction. Well, let's examine the meaning of the word *malnutrition*.

Malnutrition is the condition resulting from consuming an unbalanced diet that lacks certain nutrients.

Malnutrition is the result of an inadequate caloric intake, and it also includes nutrient deficiencies, such as necessary vitamins, minerals, and enzymes that are found in whole foods. Modern malnutrition—or what should more appropriately be called dysnutrition, for dysfunctional nutrition—is caused by the excessive caloric intake of nutrient deficient foods. These are what I like to call dead foods. According to Mark Hyman, MD, "Americans are overfed and undernourished." Dr. Hyman is a family physician who specializes in functional medicine. Functional medicine combines the philosophy of balance and restoring functions from Chinese medicine and the knowledge of biochemistry and physiology from Western medicine with the latest scientific research about how our genetics, environment, and lifestyle interact to affect our health potential. Functional medicine focuses primarily on discovering the underlying causes of chronic disease, instead of merely suppressing the symptoms. Dr. Hyman is chairman of the Institute for Functional Medicine, and he received the Linus Pauling Award for leadership in functional medicine in 2009. He also serves on the Medical Advisory Board at the *Dr. Oz Show*.

After reviewing forty years of major nutritional research and performing nutritional testing on more than ten thousand of his own patients, Dr. Hyman found that **Americans are suffering from massive nutritional deficiencies**. He went on to report that greater than 30 percent of American diets were lacking in plant-derived nutrients like magnesium, vitamin C, vitamin E, and vitamin A. He also revealed that more than 80 percent of Americans are vitamin D deficient. Shockingly, nine out of ten people are deficient in omega-3 fatty acids, or EFAs. These particular EFAs are critical for staving off inflammation, controlling blood sugar levels, and repairing nerves.

The World Health Organization cites malnutrition as the greatest single threat to the world's public health. A 2009 study published in the *Archives of Internal Medicine* further supports Dr. Hyman's findings, revealing that more than 75 percent of Americans are deficient in vitamin D. Vitamin D is instrumental in proper muscle and nerve function. **A lack of vitamin D can cause nerves to become irritated and inflamed.** Most importantly, vitamin D is necessary for your body to absorb calcium from food. We've previously seen how decreased calcium levels can cause improper firing of your peripheral nerves. In a land of abundance, let's examine how malnutrition occurs.

America's Love Affair with Processed Food

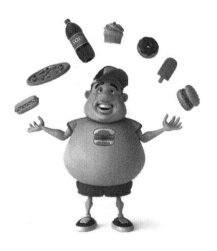

Processed foods are pervasive in this country. These include any food that comes in bags, cans, jars, or boxes. Processed foods might be fresh foods that have gone through various processing methods, such as canning, freezing, or dehydrating. Unlike healthy and fresh foods, which contain many nutrients, such as vitamins, minerals, fiber, enzymes, and healthy fats, processed foods often contain a long list of ingredients on the label. Many of the ingredients are unrecognizable, unpronounceable, and downright unhealthy. Most processed foods are laden with sweeteners, which cause insulin resistance and ultimately diabetes, artificial sweeteners, processed salt (not to be confused with natural, healthy sea salt, which is abundant in trace minerals), and artificial flavors. These so-called foods are then further saddled with hydrogenated fats, coloring, emulsifiers, hardeners, softeners, and multiple chemicals that are used to preserve the food so that they will have a longer shelf life. The texture is also altered so that these foods are more pleasing. Why is so much garbage added to what once started out as a perfectly healthy food? The reality is that the food industry substitutes healthy nutrients with addictive, flavor enhancing chemicals that are proven to harm your health, at a fraction of the cost. The consequences to the consumers are any myriad of illnesses from obesity, heart disease, diabetes, and cancer.

Seven percent of the US population eats at McDonald's daily, while an additional 20 to 25 percent eat at other fast-food venues. Thirty percent of our children between the ages of four and nineteen eat fast food on any given day. Steven Gortmaker, professor of human development and health at the Harvard School of Public Health, reported this. Americans eat 31 percent more processed food than fresh food, a statistic that is higher than any other country. Processed food comes from fast-food restaurants and also from grocery stores. Trek down the vast row of center aisles and you will find a wide variety of prepackaged foods and snacks. In fact, 90 percent of the money spent by Americans on food is spent on processed food. These processed foods are overloaded with high fructose corn syrup, artificial sweeteners, hydrogenated oils, trans fats, and neurotoxic chemicals that are used as flavor enhancers and carcinogenic food preservatives. These industrialized by-products masquerading as food are devoid of nutrients and minerals, and they are abundantly high in empty calories in the form of sugar, starch, and fat. These foods have taken the place of nutrient-rich, whole foods because they are convenient and relatively inexpensive. Your great-grandmother would not recognize the vast majority of foods filling the center aisles of grocery stores today. The processed food industry sold over $174 billion worth of fabricated, artificial food, snacks, and drinks. The outcome of all this is that America is plagued by obesity and chronic disease.

In 2007, the Johns Hopkins Bloomberg School of Public Health warned that "if not halted, the ever-increasing obesity crisis will explode by 2015 to 24 percent of children and adolescents being overweight or obese and 75 percent of adults being overweight with 41 percent being obese. One can clearly see that we are well on our way to fulfilling this statistical quota. The CDC and NIH have estimated that over twenty-one million people suffer from either prediabetes or diabetes. They go further to say that they estimate that nearly one third of our population might be undiagnosed. The World Health Organization (WHO) says that processed foods are to blame for the drastic rise in obesity, diabetes, and chronic illness that is being seen in the US and around the world. Many of these illnesses result from the obesity crisis and are due to our love affair with processed foods. So stop blaming your family genetics for your diabetes. As Dr. Oz, the popular television personality, states, "Your genetics load the gun but it is your lifestyle that pulls the trigger."

Refining Kills Nutrients

In the beginning, grains were refined to reduce insect infestation and to help preserve food longer. The process of refining became popular in the early 1900s as a way of making food more pure. Don't get excited just yet. This is not as good as it sounds. This has nothing to do with the quality of food; it has to do with the esthetics.

> Only 25% of the nutrients lost in the refining process are replaced in Enriched foods – leaving the food devoid of over 75% of its original nutrients.

Refining food makes it visually more pleasing. The process of refining yields a product with uniform texture and color. Not surprisingly, during the process of *prettifying* your food, it is essentially stripped of valuable nutrients and fiber. For example, let's look at whole grain wheat. Whole grains are made up of three parts: the bran, the germ, and the kernel. Most of the nutrients of the grain, in this case wheat grain, are stored in the bran and the germ. The germ is a rich source of minerals such as iron, calcium, B vitamins, vitamin E, protein, and good fat. The bran, which makes up the outer coating of the grain, is rich in niacin, minerals, and fiber. The process of refining whole grain wheat flour into white flour reduces the fiber content by 80 percent. Refining decimates the levels of phytonutrients, vitamins, and essential minerals. The stripped-down food is so low in quality and nutrition that the food manufacturers had to add back in synthetic vitamins, which they now refer to as enriching your food. Well, if the food were never impoverished in the first place, there would be no need for this so-called enrichment. You might think that this isn't a big deal, because at least they are putting the vitamins and minerals back, even if they are synthetic. Unfortunately, nothing could be further from the truth.

> *God, in His infinite wisdom, neglected nothing and if we would eat our food without trying to improve, change, or refine it, thereby destroying its life-giving elements, it would meet all requirements of the body.*
>
> Jethro Kloss,
> Author of *Back to Eden*
> 1863–1946

When brown rice is refined to white rice for instance, the following nutrients are destroyed: 80 percent of vitamin B-1, 67 percent of B-3, 90 percent of B-6, 80 percent of magnesium, 87 percent of zinc, 88 percent of manganese, 87 percent chromium, 60 percent of iron, 50 percent of cobalt and phosphorous, and all of the fiber and essential fatty acids (omega 3 and 6). Therefore, fully refined and polished white rice must be enriched with vitamins B-1, B-3, and iron. However, there are at least eleven nutrients lost in this process that are never replaced, even with the enrichment. Manganese, one of the lost trace minerals, is involved in the synthesis of fatty acids, which are important for the health of your nervous system. Are you beginning to see the connection yet? What you might not also realize is that certain enzymes and cofactors are present in whole foods, such as brown rice. These enzymes and cofactors allow your cells to assimilate the vitamins and minerals. You can replace the vitamins with synthetics, but you can't replace the enzymes and cofactors. So what does that mean for you? It means a lower grade of incomplete B-vitamins that your cells can't fully utilize.

Industrial Farming is Affecting Your Health

Soil Depletion and Crop Yields

Commercially grown vegetables, fruits, and grains that we eat each day are significantly less nutritious than these same foods were one hundred years ago or even just fifty years ago. Previously, it was believed that the organic farming movement was merely embellishing and using this information as a marketing ploy; however, when reports came in –revealing the decreased nutritional value of farm raised produce–it was proven to be factual. We now have solid, scientific evidence of this troubling trend, which was published in the *Journal of the American College of Nutrition* and backed up by data compiled by the USDA.

Our food is less nutritious because of industrial farming. Humans have been farming for over ten thousand years. We used to have a multitude of small family farms that produced a variety of healthful, wholesome, nutrient-rich foods. This all changed after World War II, when we started to industrial-

---

Vitamin Deficiencies

According to Centers for Disease Control and Prevention (CDC) and researchers at Tufts University, Americans are deficient in the following vitamins:

- **Vitamin E**—*93 percent deficient;*
- **Magnesium**—*56 percent deficient;*
- **Vitamin C**—*31 percent deficient;*
- **Zinc**—*12 percent deficient;*
- **B12**—*40 percent deficient;*
- **Calcium**—*68 percent deficient;*
- **B6 and vitamin D**—*75 percent deficient.*

ize the way we farm. With this type of farming method, the farm was turned into a factory operation with the end objective being to increase yields while controlling costs (i.e., the company's cost to increase their profit margin). This sounds smart and efficient, until you take a look at the toll it takes on both food quality and the environment. We replaced sound farming techniques, which yielded nutrient-dense foods, with multibillion-dollar corporations that exploit the application of science and engineering. They alter every step in the life cycle of the crop or animal to increase the company's profitability, while decreasing the individual's health.

These modern farming methods—or what should really be called corporate farming methods—depend on a large volume of synthetic and toxic fertilizers and pesticides. Studies by the EPA have shown that these chemicals strip our soils of balanced minerals and pollute and contaminate our water supplies.

The evidence indicates that our nutrient-depleted crops are suffering from what is called the environmental dilution effect. Researchers since the 1940s have understood that increases in crop yield—which were brought about by chemical fertilization, irrigation, and other means used in industrial farming—tend to decrease the concentrations of minerals in the plants and the soil. Our ancestors from a hundred years ago used manure and compost exclusively for fertilizer. Manure is nutrient rich and it serves as an excellent fertilizer, since it contains nitrogen, phosphorus, potassium, and other nutrients. Manure also adds organic matter (natural carbon compounds) to the soil, which has been shown to increase biological activity, improve soil structure, aeration, soil moisture-holding capacity, and water infiltration. Today, even in conventional farming, we have replaced manure with *superphosphate fertilizers.* These contain mainly nitrogen, potassium, and phosphorus, but they are extremely deficient in the trace minerals, such as copper, zinc and boron, to name just a few. Industrial farmers, or what we more commonly refer to as conventional farmers, like superphosphates because they act as growth stimulants.

This technique of farming produces higher crop yields, but it depletes the soil and the crops of vital minerals and nutrients. The consumers get to reap the benefits with less expensive food, but remember, "You get what you pay for!" What is the long-term cost? We get lower food quality and poor health.

The result of all of this is that most vegetables harvested today have far fewer nutrients than those from just two generations ago. One of the largest and most compelling studies on this topic was published in 2004 in the *Journal of the American College of Nutrition*. A team of scientists looked at the nutrient content of forty-three fruits and vegetables—everything from rutabaga to honeydew—grown in 1950, and they compared them to the identical fruits and veggies grown in 1999, using data from the USDA's archives. Their findings were disturbing. Levels of calcium were down 16 percent, iron was down 15 percent, and vitamin C was down 20 percent. As we examine specific plant and vegetable quality, the study further reveals the following:

- Between 1938–1990 wheat and barley: protein concentration declined by 30–50 percent.
- Between 1900–2003 wheat varieties: there was a 22–29 percent decline of six vital minerals.
- Between 1920–2001 corn (forty-five varieties): protein concentration, EFAs, amino acids significantly declined;

- Between 1950–1999 fruits and vegetables: calcium declined by 16 percent, iron declined by 15 percent, and vitamin C declined by 20 percent.
- In 1950 calcium content of broccoli averaged 12.9 mg/gram of dry weight; 2003 broccoli only averaged 4.4mg/g dry weight.

In another study involving the use of phosphorous fertilizer on raspberries, it was found that the phosphorous fertilizer caused the yield of raspberries to double, along with the levels of phosphorous; meanwhile, the levels of eight other minerals declined by 20–55 percent. Overall, when we look back over crops and their nutrient content in the past fifty years, not a single nutrient had increased.

> *"You can trace every sickness, every disease, and every ailment to a mineral deficiency."*
>
> Linus Pauling, PhD
> (Two-time Nobel Prize winner)

Because those foods contain fewer nutrients, vitamins, and minerals, the servings we do consume don't deliver as much nutrition as they once did. Fewer nutrients means lowered immunity and increased vulnerability to chronic disease and obesity. When your body doesn't get the right nutrition, it just keeps asking for more food, creating an endless cycle of cravings. What we do is misinterpret these cravings and substitute processed sugar-laden foods for whole foods. The result is that people are eating more but still not feeling satisfied. They are getting fatter and sicker without understanding the rhyme or reason. It is a proverbial nightmare from which they can't escape.

Pesticides and Herbicides and Fungicides...*Oh Crap!*

In nature, farms, vegetable gardens, or flower gardens can be plagued with pests. These pests may come in the form of weeds, which can compete and take over the land on which you are attempting to grow your fruits, vegetables, or flowerbed. Or they may come in the form of various insects that enjoy feeding on your plants and causing damage. A pest can also take the form of a fungus that infects plants. To combat this infiltration, we have grown accustomed to using potent chemicals to eradicate these pesky problems. Pesticide is a broad term used to describe three types of chemical agents:

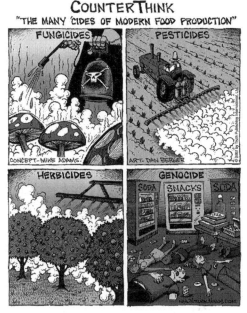

Concept by Mike Adams, art by Dan Berger www.naturalnews.com

1. Insecticides—used to kill insects (industrial and household);
2. Herbicides—used to kill weeds or undesirable plants (industrial and lawn);
3. Fungicides—used to control fungi that cause fungal diseases in plants.

We've mentioned outdoor uses for pesticides, which are commonly used on an industrial level, but let's not forget the common household pesticides that lurk in the majority of kitchen cabinets. Let's take a look at what we can find in an average kitchen:

- cockroach and ant killer (sprays and baits);
- insect repellant sprays for bodily use;
- flea and tick sprays, powders, and pet collars;
- kitchen and bath disinfectants to kill mold and mildew (fungus);
- lawn and garden products (weed killer and fire ant killer).

In the United States, hundreds of millions of pounds of pesticides are sprayed annually. Over 95 percent of sprayed insecticides and herbicides reach destinations other than their target. These chemicals contaminate the air, water supplies, topsoil, bottom sediments, and food. If that isn't bad enough, we use these chemicals within the closed environment of our home, and insanely enough, we spray these toxic chemicals (to ward off mosquitoes and other biting insects) directly onto our skin, as if they're cologne. We would never dream of whipping out a can of Raid and spraying it directly on our body, but through the ploy of clever marketing, we have been brainwashed into believing that topical bug sprays or lotions are different. It is estimated that more than ten thousand people suffer from acute pesticide poisoning every year, as reported by the CDC. It's also estimated that many more people suffer the adverse effects of pesticide poisoning without reporting their illness. Although the EPA finally banned DDT in 1972 after three decades of use, the public is not aware that the newer pesticides that have emerged are even more dangerous.

Pesticides enter our body through direct contact, like walking or golfing on a beautiful green lawn that has been sprayed with herbicides, and eating conventional, non-organic foods that have been sprayed with these chemicals. I want to dispel the myth that washing your produce gets rid of pesticides. This simply is not true. You may indeed be able to wash off pesticide residue on the outer surface of your fruits and vegetables; however, these chemicals become an integrated part of the food, both internally and externally, since they have been grown in chemical-laden soil, from which they extract their nutrients.

Here are the latent problems with these chemicals: they add to the toxic burden within our body. Some contain lead, mercury, and arsenic. This heavy metal burden requires extra minerals from an already mineral-deficient body to minimize the damage to our cells. As such, it sends our body further into nutrient depletion. Pesticides are also carcinogenic and linked with a number of cancers, including leukemia. On top of this, scientists have discovered that some pesticides can both mimic and compete with hormones such as thyroid, estrogen, and testosterone, to name a few. As a result, they can displace and interfere with the functions of these hormones, creating a hormonal imbalance. If that were not bad enough, **pesticides, especially organophosphates, cause damage and disruption to the nervous system.**

The results of a study in 2006 led by the University of North Dakota's Energy and Environmental Research Center (EERC) and funded by the impartial CDC (Centers For Disease Control and Prevention) has linked pesticide exposure to neurological diseases.

This study showed neurological changes resulting from pesticides associated with Parkinson's disease, multiple sclerosis, epilepsy and Alzheimer's. These findings were consistent with a study performed by Harvard School of Public Health in 2006. Other studies have shown a direct correlation with pesticide organophosphate levels and peripheral neuropathy. The organophosphate disrupts activity at the synaptic junction.

> "Studies have shown a direct correlation with pesticide organophosphate levels and peripheral neuropathy."
>
> Harvard School of Public Health Study, 2006

We have previously discussed how pesticides can mimic hormones. When a pesticide is introduced into the body, it can mimic acetylcholine. Acetylcholine is a neurotransmitter that is used in the peripheral nervous system to stimulate muscle fiber activity and contraction. In the autonomic nervous system, it regulates smooth muscle and cardiac muscle function. Acetylcholine is released into the neuron. It then crosses the gap to signal the next neuron to fire. In the peripheral nervous system, this signaling tells the nerve to fire to initiate muscle contraction; however, after the nerve fires- the acetylcholine must be broken down. If it were allowed to linger, it would create a repeated, uncontrolled firing of the neuron, resulting in nerve death. An enzyme called acetylcholinesterase must break down the acetylcholine. When an organophosphate pesticide enters the body, it mimics acetylcholine. The problem occurs because acetylcholinesterase cannot break down the organophosphates. As a result, it cannot prevent the neuron from firing. This can lead to peripheral neuropathy, and in more extreme cases it can lead to convulsions and seizures.

It is of the utmost importance for you and your loved ones to reduce your exposure to pesticides. There are many natural and less expensive alternatives to control pests inside and outside of your home. For topical bug spray, I use Burt's Bees herbal insect repellant and Badger anti-bug spray. They are all natural, safe, and highly effective. Their ingredients are blends of rosemary, lemongrass, citronella, and other essential oils. Now, doesn't this sound much better than spraying yourself with chemicals like Diethyl-meta-Toluamide (DEET) and Picaridin?

> *True health care reform cannot happen in Washington. By cleansing your body on a regular basis and eliminating as many toxins as possible from your environment, your body can begin to heal itself, prevent disease, and become stronger and more resilient than you ever dreamed possible!*
>
> Dr. Edward Group III

8

NUTRIENTS TO HEAL NERVES

"The human body heals itself and nutrition provides the resources to accomplish the task."

Roger Williams, PhD

By now you have learned that like all other parts of your body, nerves undergo a continual process of maintenance and repair. For a nerve to remain healthy or for repair to occur over a damaged area of the nerve, it must have an ongoing supply of good quality nutrients. Scientific research has established that many vitamins, minerals, and herbs are strong weapons against nerve damage, and they are irrefutably necessary for nerve repair and healing. Let's examine some of these nutrients.

Antioxidants

Many people have heard the term *antioxidant,* but few people actually know what it is or how it works. Antioxidants are

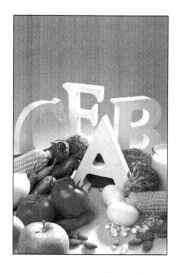

nutrients—like vitamins, minerals, and enzymes—that function to prevent damage from occurring to the cells within your body or to repair the damage that has already been done. An antioxidant accomplishes this by slowing cellular oxidation, which is a naturally occurring process in nature and in our bodies. For example, a banana will turn brown—as will any fruit, like apples or pears—when it's been cut into. Leave that bowl of delicious guacamole uncovered on the counter, and it goes from a festive green color to a disgusting brown color in just a few minutes. An old nail will become rusty with time. A paper cut on your skin will become inflamed. These are all examples of oxidation.

As oxygen interacts with any type of cell in your body, it produces a change. Sometimes this change is as normal as cells dying off to be replaced by new cells. This is what happens when our old, dead skin falls off. The birth and death of cells in the body is an ongoing, necessary process that makes oxidation a normal process of cellular function. However, there is a downside to oxidation. Although the body is very efficient at metabolizing oxygen for critical functions, approximately 1–2 percent of the cells will become damaged in the process, causing free radicals to form. A free radical is a damaged cell that is missing a critical molecule, such as an electron. This cell will now go on a rampage to steal an electron from another molecule, damaging or killing the other molecule in the process. The problem with free radicals is not that they simply kill off other molecules in the body; they actually damage the DNA within the cell.

When a cell's DNA gets damaged, that cell becomes mutated. Then, when the cell replicates, as it normally does, the mutation will be replicated. Damaged free radicals set off a chain reaction similar to a series of dominoes falling down. This sets the stage for chronic disease and neurodegeneration.

Increased oxidative stress creates large amounts of free radicals, which can cause destruction to peripheral nerves. Another important factor in the oxidation process is that neurons are one of the few cells that don't require insulin to get glucose into the nerve cells. As a result, people with elevated blood sugar levels accumulate excess glucose within the nerves, which is then converted to sorbitol. Sorbitol is a big culprit in causing free radical damage to the nerve.

Oxidative stress occurs from a constant chemical assault by environmental toxins and the foods that we eat. It even results from the chronic, persistent barrage of emotional stress that we encounter daily. So, how do we combat all of the free radicals that occur within the body? We do so with the help of antioxidants. Researcher and professor of nutrition at Tufts University in Boston, Jeffrey Blumberg, PhD, states, "Toxins are ubiquitous in the environment. The oxidative burden on the body is much, much, much higher than it was two hundred years ago. It's a fact of modern life that we have to take into consideration. In the twenty-first century, people need to get more antioxidants

Foods High in Antioxidants
- blueberries
- cranberries
- elderberries
- strawberries
- blackberries
- raisins
- acai berries
- prunes
- spinach
- kale
- raw cocoa bean

in their diet to offset all of these assaults." Antioxidants work to stop the damaging chain reaction started by free radicals. The role of the antioxidants is to either prevent the chain reaction from occurring or to halt it, if it has already begun. Unfortunately, in the twenty-first century, it is impossible to get all of the necessary antioxidants that you need from diet alone. It doesn't matter if you follow a Mediterranean diet, a macrobiotic diet, or a vegan diet. It is simply impossible. Let's familiarize you with some of the various antioxidants, especially the ones that play a significant role with nerve repair.

Alpha-lipoic acid

Alpha-lipoic acid (ALA) is a powerful antioxidant that assists in converting glucose into energy. It also plays a significant role in lowering blood sugar levels, thus regulating glucose metabolism and improving insulin sensitivity. In the section on diabetes, we mentioned that insulin escorts glucose into the cell. A very interesting fact about ALA is that it can transport glucose into your cells independent of insulin. If this isn't exciting enough, you might also like to know that ALA also increases the efficiency of insulin. As such, it slows or prevents the onset of diabetes. ALA has been shown to protect the heart and the kidneys, and the small blood vessels that are responsible for microcirculation in the extremities.

Every cell utilizes ALA, and it is both fat- and water-soluble. Therefore, it is effective in either a fat or a water medium in the body.

> Alpha-lipoic acid aids in nerve repair by escalating the speed of conduction, thus improving communication and proper signaling of muscle fibers.

Everyone on this planet requires antioxidant protection, but this is especially the case with diabetics. They require a stronger source of protection than a healthy individual, and ALA fulfills this need. It has a substantial ability to squelch free radicals and aid the liver in the detoxification process. ALA's ability to restore vitamin C and E levels, two other important antioxidants in nerve repair, is particularly significant.

ALA aids in nerve repair by escalating the speed of conduction. This improves nerve communication and enables the proper signaling and stimulation of muscle fibers. As a result of this, muscular atrophy, or wasting, is slowed and in some cases halted. Other notable actions of ALA are its ability to boost circulation, allowing for increased oxygenation and the delivery of nutrients to the nerve cells. The added benefit of enhanced circulation is that cellular toxins and wastes will be flushed away, as opposed to becoming stagnant within the tissues and vessels. The end result is improved microcirculation within the capillaries in your legs, hands, eyes, heart, and brain.

Interestingly, doctors in Germany have been prescribing alpha-lipoic acid for decades to help patients with type 2 diabetes and to prevent diabetes-related neuropathy. The research has shown that ALA is helpful in treating diabetic neuropathy, and the evidence has also revealed that it is equally effective with CIPN (chemotherapy induced peripheral neuropathy), according to a study performed in Austria. Aside from aiding in nerve repair for sensorimotor polyneuropathy, alpha-lipoic acid has been found to be effective in healing autonomic neuropathy. It has been shown to help normalize fluctuating heart rates, especially in diabetics, by repairing the damaged nerves of the heart.

Alpha-lipoic acid is made in only minute amounts within the body. Therefore, you must consume it from your diet and supplementation. Foods that contain this antioxidant include spinach, broccoli, beef, brewer's yeast, and certain organ meats, such as kidney and heart. It's safe to assume that the percentage of people consuming organ meats on a regular basis is extremely small. It is equally important to remember that due to the decreased nutrient content in today's food supplies, it will be extremely difficult—if not impossible—to acquire therapeutic dosages of alpha-lipoic acid in one's diet. For this reason, I always prescribe alpha-lipoic acid supplements for all of my patients with neuropathy. A therapeutic dosage for nerve repair is 600 mg taken twice a day.

Vitamin C

Vitamin C, or ascorbic acid, is a water-soluble vitamin. We do not have the capability of producing vitamin C within our body; therefore, we are dependent upon our diet and supplementation to get the necessary levels of vitamin C. New evidence shows that vitamin C plays a crucial role in protecting nerve cells from oxidative damage.

Scientists at Stanford University have found that vitamin C has strong antioxidant properties, and it is able to neutralize free radicals. Once inside the body, vitamin C will change from ascorbic acid to ascorbate. In this form, it has the ability to donate its own electrons to free radicals to stop their rampage. In doing this, ascorbate protects other components of the cell, like its DNA and proteins, from further oxidizing and mutating. Excessive oxidative damage can lead to nerve cell death. Researchers also noted that vitamin C is prevalent in certain areas of the brain, as well as between nerve cells. Vitamin C works as a natural anti-inflammatory, helping protect and restore the myelin sheath of a nerve. Their studies have effectively shown vitamin C's capability in repairing and preventing nerve damage. The therapeutic dosage for vitamin C is 2500 mg.

Vitamin E

Vitamin E is an essential fat-soluble vitamin. This means that it is necessary for the proper function of all of your cells. It is also a very potent antioxidant. Vitamin E occurs in two forms: tocopherol and tocotrienol. In both of these forms, vitamin E exists in four different states: alpha, beta, gamma, and delta. Each form, tocopherol and tocotrienol, has varying advantages. Tocotrienols are your natural sources of vitamin E. They are found 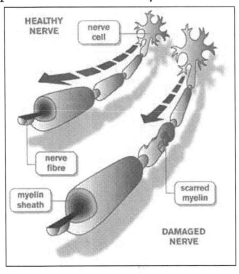 in food sources such as wheat germ, barley, oats, rye, rice, bran, and saw palmetto. The benefit of the tocotrienols is that they are assimilated into the cell membrane with greater ease and availability. Tocopherols are a synthetic form of vitamin E, which means that they are typically created in a laboratory. It is possible to find some naturally occurring tocopherol in palm oil, safflower oil, peanut oil, soybean oil, cocoa butter, rice bran, and wheat germ. However the vast majority of vitamin E supplements contain synthetic tocopherols. The most commonly used form of tocopherol is alpha tocopherol. Alpha tocopherol has the highest vitamin E activity. To explore the effect that vitamin E has on neuropathy, we will focus on alpha-tocopherol.

Vitamin E plays a critical role in maintaining normal nerve function. It has been shown that people who have low levels of vitamin E in their body frequently suffer from nerve dysfunction, including nerve damage and neuropathy.

As a powerful antioxidant, vitamin E can prevent or even reverse the effects of free radicals, which are produced at a very high rate in nerves. This plays a significant role in your peripheral nerve health. Vitamin E protects the membranes of the nerve cells. As you will recall, most of the peripheral nervous system is myelinated with neurons that are rich in layers of lipids (fats). This is the main component of the myelin sheath. Since Vitamin E is a fat-soluble vitamin, it can pass into the nerve membranes quite easily, thus squelching the destructive free radicals. Without essential levels of vitamin E in the body, the demyelination of the neurons can occur, leading to slow nerve conduction, poor muscle function, and sensory problems. For this reason, with vitamin E deficiency, the toxins in the body damage the membranes of the nerves. Recent studies suggest that low vitamin E content in the nerves is indicative of developing nerve degeneration. Demyelinating neuropathy, a condition in which the myelin sheath is scarred or destroyed, has been observed in conjunction with vitamin E deficiencies. As a result, peripheral neuropathy ensues.

The *American Family Physician* journal, reports that vitamin E deficiency most frequently affects the sensory nerves, leading to symptoms like numbness and tingling. Demyelinating neuropathy has also been seen with vitamin E deficiency. In this situation, the substance covering the nerve, myelin, is destroyed. This leads to slow nerve conduction, and it can cause muscle function and sensory problems.

Although alpha-tocopherol is the most familiar and publicized form in the commercial industry, it is critical to realize that alpha-tocopherol is not the end-all in the vitamin E family. When trying to prevent cardiovascular disease, the form of vitamin E that you want to use is the tocotrienols. However, since this book focuses on healing neuropathy, we have focused on the most active form of vitamin E that accomplishes this: alpha-tocopherol.

Vitamin E is one of the least toxic fat-soluble vitamins, making it safe even when administered orally in dosages up to 2000 mg or IU (international units) per day. Caution should be exercised by anyone taking vitamin E who is deficient in vitamin K (the vitamin necessary for normal clotting) or who is taking anticoagulant medications.

N-acetylcysteine (NAC)

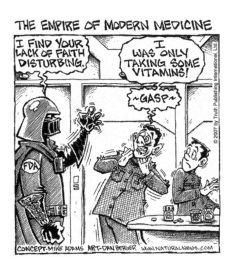

N-acetylcysteine (NAC) is an amino acid with potent antioxidant effects. It is a precursor to glutathione, an intrinsic and potent antioxidant. The lymphocytes (immune cells in the lymph tissue) and the liver use it to detoxify chemicals and other toxins introduced into the body. It has been shown to be highly effective in detoxifying environmental pollutants, heavy metals, tobacco smoke, and alcohol, all of which play a role in nerve damage. Research studies have shown that NAC, through a series of complicated interactions, inhibits the development of functional and structural abnormalities of the peripheral nerve. Further animal studies have shown that NAC can inhibit diabetic neuropathy and protect against neuropathies caused by chemotherapy drugs. NAC has even been shown to reduce nausea in chemotherapy patients.

Gamma Linoleic Acid (GLA)

GLA is an essential omega-6 fatty acid that your body must get from dietary sources for proper health. For the last twenty years, research has demonstrated that natural sources of GLA supplementation play a large role in preventing and improving neuropathy. According to the University of Maryland Medical Center, GLA is important for many physiological functions. In particular, GLA aids with diminishing symptoms of diabetic neuropathy. Our body utilizes GLA for building healthy nerve structure and maintaining healthy nerve function.

A healthy body can manufacture gamma linoleic acid from linoleic acid, which is commonly found in vegetable oils, such as flaxseed oil, safflower oil, sunflower oil, corn oil, soybean oil, and canola oil. However, not all of these oils, such as corn, soybean, and canola, are healthy choices for oils. Also, bear in mind that I mentioned that a healthy body can make this conversion. It's been my experience that people who have not been diagnosed with a medical condition consider themselves to be healthy. I know that a lot of obese individuals have not yet been diagnosed with any conditions or illnesses, but I assure you they are far from healthy. Although these people may be lovely people, an absence of diagnostic findings on lab work doesn't mean that the turbulence isn't brewing under the surface. However, for the sake of expediency, let's take a look at obvious conditions in which we would expect to find impaired conversion of linoleic acid to gamma linoleic acid. Can you guess one obvious one? We've mentioned it continually throughout this book. If you guessed, diabetes, you are absolutely correct! However, it doesn't simply start with diabetes. Actually, any type of glucose intolerance, like that which is found in metabolic syndrome, insulin resistance, and prediabetes prohibits this conversion. This will result in lower levels of GLA and its metabolites in the tissue. Other conditions that would inhibit GLA conversion are digestive disorders, such as indigestion, acid reflux, GERD, IBS, and inflammatory bowel disorders. So, for the vast majority of the population, GLA must be supplied through dietary supplementation.

A good source of gamma linoleic acid is found in oils such as borage oil, evening primrose oil, and black currant seed oil. All of these things are what we consider to be good oils, which means that they have a vast array of health benefits. The main difference between the three oils is the amount of GLA that they each contain. Borage oil has the highest concentration of GLA. It is made up of 23 percent gamma linoleic acid. Black currant seed oil contains 15–17 percent gamma linoleic acid and evening primrose oil contains 8–10 percent. In clinical research, all three of these oils have been found to be effective in treating polyneuropathy. As a matter of fact, research studies from 1986 to the present day have found GLA supplementation to be highly efficacious. These studies have consistently concluded that both pain diminution and nerve restoration were accomplished with the use of GLA. This was verified and corroborated by measuring peripheral nerve function, nerve conduction velocity, nerve capillary blood flow, hot and cold thresholds, sensation, reflexes, and muscle strength. Later laboratory studies found that GLA was even more effective when used in conjunction with antioxidants—especially vitamin C.

Acetyl-L-carnitine (ALC)

Acetyl-L-carnitine (ALC) is a well-researched nutritional supplement that is synthesized to provide a more bioavailable form of L-carnitine, Acetyl-L-carnitine functions as an antioxidant and promotes the production of glutathione, which is considered to be the master antioxidant in cells.

ALC is proven to have neuroprotective properties. It expedites nerve regeneration, improves nerve conduction velocity—the speed of signal transmission—and it prevents and slows down the onset and development of cardiac neuropathy in diabetics. Two recent studies have found that acetyl-L-carnitine can limit the neuropathy associated with some chemotherapy drugs, as well as, diabetes. In two related studies of diabetic nerve degeneration and neuropathy, acetyl-L-carnitine accelerated nerve regeneration in an experimental study in which the researchers simulated a nerve injury.

All of the studies demonstrate that ALC treatment is efficacious in alleviating symptoms, particularly pain, and it improves nerve fiber regeneration and vibration perception in patients with established diabetic neuropathy.

Omega 3s

Omega-3 fatty acids are essential fatty acids: they are absolutely necessary for many functions within cells and organs. However, the body can't make them. The only way for you to get omega-3 fatty acids is through food or supplementation. Omega-3s are commonly found in fish, especially cold-water varieties such as salmon, sardines, anchovies, tuna, and halibut, or in other seafood, such as algae and krill. Some plants, seeds, and nuts, also, contain omega-3s. We discussed in a previous chapter the rising rates of heavy metal and other contaminants in fish, so you must be careful about the amount of fish that you consume.

Also known as polyunsaturated fatty acids (PUFAs), omega-3 fatty acids play a crucial role in brain function, as well as normal growth and development. They have also gained notice because they have been shown to reduce the risk of heart disease and are widely consumed for their anti-inflammatory powers. Omega-3s are crucial components of cell membranes, including the delicate myelin sheath that protects nerves.

Inflammation plays a significant role in nerve damage, especially in the peripheral nervous system. Inflammation is a normal part of the healing process. When you cut yourself, your body will produce inflammatory exudates to heal the wound. Once the wound is healed, the inflammation will stop. The problem ensues when this normal process runs amok and it doesn't turn off. This occurs in response to

> **Omega-3 fats help prevent nerve damage and assist the repair process**

constant mental or emotional stress, poor diet, lack of exercise, hidden allergens from food or the environment, chronic exposure to toxins like mercury and pesticides, and exposure to mold and seasonal allergens. These factors will cause the inflammatory cycle to run constantly. After a while, this inflammation will begin to inhibit proper organ function, and it will also cause nerve damage.

Both the central and peripheral nervous systems rely on omega-3 fatty acids for normal function and repair. According to a 2007 study published in the *Journal of Prostaglandins, Leukotrienes, and Essential Fatty Acids*, omega-3 fatty acids can help regenerate nerve tissue following an injury to the nervous system. This research also demonstrated that omega-3s can have neuroprotective effects against spinal cord injury.

DHA, an important part of the omega-3 family, was found to improve recovery from spinal cord injuries, according to a study published in the October 2010 issue of the *Journal of Neurotrauma*. In the laboratory animal study, results showed improved nerve function within the first week. By week six of DHA supplementation, a reduction was found in myelin and nerve fiber damage. Researchers concluded, "DHA shows substantial potential to protect the spinal cord from damage."

A more recent study carried out at Queen Mary University of London revealed that omega-3 fatty acids have the ability to protect nerves from injury, and they help nerves regenerate. Omega-3s have been effective in both direct injury to the nerves and indirect injuries, such as chronic inflammatory reactions.

This new study, which was published in the January 2012 issue of the Journal of Neuroscience, suggests that omega-3s play a significant role in speeding recovery from nerve injury.

Interestingly enough, the study focused on peripheral nerve cells.

Studies have shown that omega-3 fatty acids are able to reduce demyelination in the nerves of diabetic animals, which reduces neuropathic pain.

Fish Oil vs. Flaxseed Oil

As we discussed, you can acquire your omega-3 fatty acids by either consuming food or supplements. To achieve a therapeutic dosage of omega-3s, approximately 4000 mg, you would need to consume a boatload of fish daily, which is not recommend due to the chemical contaminants in fish. Levels of contamination vary by species and locale, and whether the fish are wild or farmed. In recent years, farmed salmon has been shown to contain more toxic chemicals than wild salmon, largely because of chemicals in the foods they are given. This makes consuming fish oil a better alternative to acquiring therapeutic levels of omega-3s.

Did You Know...

Farmed fish are far inferior to their wild counterparts:

- Farm-raised fish provide fewer omega-3 fats than wild fish.
- Farm-raised fish are doused with antibiotics.
- Farm-raised fish are exposed to more concentrated pesticides than wild fish.
- Farmed salmon, in addition, are given a salmon-colored dye in their feed, without which their flesh would be an unappetizing grey color.
- Aquafarming has a significant negative impact on wild salmon. Sea lice from fish farms kill up to 95 percent of juvenile wild salmon that migrate past them. (Krkosek M, Lewis MA. Proc. Natl. Acad. Sci. USA)

The question I'm often asked is, "What is the difference between taking fish oil or flax oil? Can't I get my omega-3s from either?"

The omega-3 fatty acids found in fish oil are vital to your good health. Unfortunately, many people have been led to believe that they'll get these same health benefits from oils like flaxseed, primrose, or borage, and this is plainly not accurate. Fish oil contains the omega-3s necessary for overall health as well as nerve function. The components of these omega fatty acids are EPA (eicosapentanoic acid) and DHA (docosahexanoic acid). EPA and DHA are the components that aid in circulatory and nerve health, and they repair many other vital cell functions. Fish oil is rich in both EPA and DHA. A vegetarian-based oil, like flaxseed, contains alpha-linoleic acid (ALA). ALA can be used to synthesize both EPA and DHA, albeit inefficiently.

According to research published in the *International Journal for Vitamin and Nutrition*, the degree of conversion of ALA is unreliable and restricted. More specifically, studies in humans have shown that whereas the conversion of high doses of ALA to EPA occurs at restricted levels, the conversion to DHA is severely restricted. The body uses various enzymes to convert ALA to other omega-3s, and the process is not very efficient, especially as one gets older. Estimates of the rate of conversion of ALA to EPA/DHA range from 5 percent to 25 percent. To make sufficient amounts of EPA and DHA, one needs to consume five or six times more ALA than relying on fish oil alone. We can now see that consumption of only flaxseed oil that contains mainly ALA is not always adequate to supply all the levels of DHA and EPA the body requires. Also, women convert ALA to EPA/DHA more efficiently than men. Healthy young women can typically convert 30 percent of ALA to EPA and DHA, whereas men may only convert 12 percent of ALA to DHA and EPA. As a final result, taking a vegetarian-based oil, like flaxseed, will not give you the same neuro-protective results as taking fish oil.

In our practice, we always recommend fish oil. However, we do not recommend just any fish oil. It is important to take cold-pressed fish oil. This maintains the integrity and quantity of EPA and DHA. Equally necessary is the distillation process to take out all of the harmful toxins present. There are two main types of distillation methods: steam distillation and molecular distillation. Both of these methods do an excellent job at removing toxins. With the process of steam distillation, you do not get as high a concentration of EPA/DHA as you do with molecular distillation, but this isn't a no-brainer. Unfortunately, in the process of molecular distillation, many companies will use the chemical hexane, a known carcinogen, to remove toxins. In my opinion, that merely sounds like you are swapping one toxin for another toxin. Ridiculous, don't you think? Hexane does not have to be used. Instead, manufacturers can use ethanol, which is much safer, to separate and filter out the toxins like mercury and PCBs, but this process is more expensive and it cuts into their bottom-line profits.

Confused yet? Don't be. Here's the lowdown. Purchase fish oil that is high in EPA/DHA, cold-pressed, and steam distilled.

(Exercise caution if taking fish oil while on warfarin; the combination may increase your risk of bleeding.)

Vitamin B-A Family Affair

The most important vitamins in nerve regeneration are the vitamin B complex family. There are a total of eight B vitamins, and they are essential for metabolism, growth, reproduction, appetite, healthy digestive tract, nervous system function, and blood cell formation.

The family of B vitamins is water-soluble, which means that the body does not store them. As such, you must use these vitamins right away. Any B vitamins not put to use will be excreted from the body through the urine. Vitamin B12 is the only water-soluble vitamin that can be stored in the liver for many years. All B vitamins help the body convert food (carbohydrates) into fuel in the form of glucose, which is used to produce energy.

Of the entire family of B vitamins, the most important players with regard to healthy nerve function, repair, and regeneration are B1, B3, B5, B6, and B12.

A German journal, *Klinische Wochenschrift*, published a study showing that B vitamins help nerve regeneration resulting from injury. In this study, vitamin B1, B6, and B12 were tested. All three vitamins had significant nerve repair and regrowth enhancing abilities.

Thiamine–B1

Thiamine (also spelled *thiamin*) is known as vitamin B1. It helps the body break down carbohydrates for energy. It is one of the eight water-soluble B vitamins that your body needs for proper nerve function. Thiamine is also involved in the production of DNA, necessary for nerve cells reproduction. A thiamine deficiency can lead to nerve damage and neurological symptoms, such as numbness in your limbs.

Certain animal studies have shown a decrease in neuropathic pain when a combination of vitamin B1, vitamin B6, and vitamin B12 were administered. Vitamin B1 can be produced in the laboratory as a fat-soluble B vitamin. This is called benfotiamine, and it has been used to treat alcoholic and diabetic neuropathies effectively. Significant results of pain relief were seen in as little as three weeks.

The best whole-food source of B1 is brewer's yeast, which contains 4.3 mg of thiamine per ounce. Other good whole food sources are:

Whole grains and legumes: Wheat germ, brown rice, rice bran, oatmeal, millet, legumes, peanuts, sunflower seeds, and dried soybeans are rich sources of vitamin B1–with sunflower seeds being the richest source, as they contain 3.3 mg of thiamine per 140 grams of seeds.

However, we never recommend eating soybeans or peanuts. Let's start with soy first. All conventional soy crops in the US are genetically engineered, unless they are organic. Soy (including soybeans) is high in phytoestrogens contributing to an elevation of the body's estrogen levels in both men and women. Because of this, soy has the capability to push you into estrogen dominance. Soy can also cause damage to your thyroid by inhibiting your uptake of iodine (a necessary nutrient for healthy thyroid function), and is extremely high in phytates. Phytates are enzyme inhibitors that block the absorption of minerals in your digestive tract. Unlike most grains or nuts, where overnight soaking breaks down the phytates, simply soaking soy–even in an acidic medium–won't do the trick. In order to receive the health benefits you often hear about, soy must be organic and fermented. If you eat soy, make sure to consume small, limited amounts and stick with fermented, organic soy products like miso, tempeh, natto or naturally fermented soy sauce–known as tamari sauce.

The average American consumes more than six pounds of peanuts and peanut butter products each year, under the illusion that it is a healthy snack. The problem with peanuts is that it is one of the most pesticide-contaminated crops. On top of that, peanuts are frequently contaminated with a carcinogenic mold called aflatoxin. Peanuts and products like peanut butter are loaded with omega 6 fats creating an imbalance between your omega 3:6 ration, when consumed in excess. If you are a *die-hard* peanut lover, there are some things that you can do to minimize the negative effects. First, switch brands of peanut butter to Arrowhead Mills organic peanut butter. Since this peanut butter is organic, the nuts have been grown free of pesticides. The peanuts used to make this brand of peanut butter are grown in New Mexico. Because the climate in this state is very dry, aflatoxins have not been reported to be a problem. Lastly, in order to reduce the omega 6 fat in the peanut butter, pour off the excess oil instead of stirring it into the peanut butter. If the peanut butter is too dry for your liking, you can stir in some melted coconut oil, olive oil (EVOO) or macadamia nut oil.

Meat and eggs: Most meat products like poultry, pork, liver, kidney, and fish are excellent sources of vitamin B1. Egg yolk is also a good source of vitamin B1. So stop throwing out the yolks, while just consuming the whites. Egg yolk is not the culprit of your high cholesterol. The problem is all of the other processed, high-fat, high-sugar foods that you are consuming. Whenever a person with high cholesterol comes to me, I remove all of the bad culprits in their diet, but I leave in whole eggs. I allow my patients to eat two to three whole eggs daily and guess what—their cholesterol levels drop even though they are still consuming eggs.

Nuts and fruits: All nuts should be raw for best nutrient content. Pistachio nuts, Brazil nuts, pecans, plums, and raisins are rich food sources of vitamin B1. High vitamin B1 content can be obtained from dry fruits if eaten dried and raw. The cooked and roasted dry fruits lose nearly 30 percent of vitamin B1.

Vegetables: Mushrooms, brussels sprouts, asparagus, peas, cabbage, broccoli, avocados, raisins, and green leafy vegetables, such as kale and mustard greens, are rich sources of vitamin B1.

Niacin–B3

Niacin, or vitamin B-3, like thiamine, helps your body metabolize energy from the food that you eat. It is involved in building, repairing, and maintaining your nervous system. Vitamin B3 helps your body repair and regenerate both skin and nerve cells. It also helps your body keep cholesterol levels normal.

In the United States, alcoholism is the main cause of vitamin B3 deficiency. A niacin deficiency is known as pellagra, and includes neurological symptoms such as headaches, fatigue, confusion, and memory loss. Niacin is found abundantly in animal products, like meat, poultry, and fish. It is also found in yeast, cereal, legumes and seeds.

The best food sources of vitamin B3 are beets, brewer's yeast, organ meats like liver and kidneys, salmon, swordfish, tuna and sunflower seeds. In addition, the body can convert tryptophan, an amino acid, into niacin. Tryptophan rich foods include poultry, red meat, eggs, and dairy products.

Pantothenic Acid–B5

Pantothenic acid is another B complex vitamin that is present in all living cells. B5 is necessary for the body to synthesize coenzyme A or CoA. This coenzyme allows the body to convert glucose into a usable form of energy needed to build and repair cells.

Pantothenic acid gets its name from the Greek root *pantos*, meaning "everywhere," because it is easily accessible in a whole-food diet and found in a wide variety of foods. Based on this, B5 deficiencies should be uncommon. However, a lot of vitamin B5 is lost during the refining process and cooking with high heat (anything cooked above 180 degrees). We also find B5 deficiencies in people consuming a highly processed diet.

Good sources of pantothenic acid include organ meats, brewer's yeast, egg yolks, fish, chicken, whole grains, cheese, peanuts, dried beans, and a variety of vegetables such as sweet potatoes, green peas, cauliflower, and avocados. Another source of B5 is the good bacterial flora in the intestines. Your good bacteria, also known as probiotics, produce vitamin B5 in your intestines. If you have been on a number of antibiotic therapies and you have never replenished your probiotics, it is very likely that you are deficient in B5.

Pantothenic acid plays a role in supporting adrenal function and steroid hormone production. Because of this, it has come to be known as the anti-stress vitamin. It supports the adrenal glands to increase the production of cortisol and other adrenal hormones to help counteract stress and enhance metabolism. Once B5 is converted to coenzyme A, it supports the synthesis of acetylcholine, an important neurotransmitter that is responsible for nerve impulse firing and neuromuscular functions. Your body needs pantothenic acid to synthesize cholesterol, which is important for the health of your neurons.

According to research conducted at the Linus Pauling Institute, vitamin B5 helps build and protect the myelin sheath, the protective covering of your nerve cells that enhances signal transmission and speed. Vitamin B5 deficiency can lead to nerve damage due to the degeneration of the myelin sheath. Humans need a minimum of five milligrams of pantothenic acid to maintain healthy nerve function. To repair nerve damage, a larger dosage is necessary.

Pyridoxine–B6

Vitamin B6 is necessary for more than one hundred enzymatic reactions in the body. It acts as a coenzyme in the breakdown and utilization of carbohydrates, fats, and proteins. It also aids in adrenal function and helps calm and maintain a healthy nervous system. Within the nervous tissue, vitamin B6 helps the nervous system send messages to and from the brain. It plays a significant role in the production of neurotransmitters, the chemicals that allow brain and nerve cells to communicate with one another. It is also important for the synthesis of lipids (fats) that are part of the myelin sheath.

B6 has also been found to reduce the major risk factors found in the development of diabetic neuropathy. In the research, patients suffering from diabetic neuropathies have been shown to have a B6 deficiency. Vitamin B6 helps repair nerves in nerve compression injuries like carpal tunnel syndrome. A vitamin B6 deficiency can lead to nerve damage in the hands and feet, which results in polyneuropathy.

Good food sources of vitamin B6 are brewer's yeast, fish, poultry, meat, beans (legumes), eggs, sunflower seeds, vegetables (especially spinach, carrots, sweet potatoes, and peas), and fruits, including bananas.

Note: If you are taking Levodopa, which is used to treat Parkinson's disease, vitamin B6 can possibly reduce the effectiveness of levodopa therapy.

Cobalamin – B12

Vitamin B12 is an especially important vitamin for maintaining healthy nerve cells. Similar to its other family members, vitamin B12 helps the body break down and use fuel from food. It also helps the body make red blood cells, and it assists in the production of DNA and RNA, the body's genetic material. It also helps the brain and spinal cord function correctly.

The natural form of B12, which is found only in animal products, is methylcobalamin. This form is the most bioavailable, which means that your cells easily utilize it. The most common forms of supplemental B12 are cyanocobalamin or hydroxycobalamin. They are synthetic and produced in the laboratory. They lack the level of bioavailability that methylcobalimin has, but they are frequently used in supplements because they are a less expensive source, which increases profitability for the manufacturer.

Vitamin B12 participates in the function, maintenance, and repair of nerve cells. It is also utilized in the production and maintenance of myelin, the protective covering of the neurons. Low levels of B12 can cause a range of symptoms, including numbness or tingling sensation in the fingers and toes, fatigue, shortness of breath, diarrhea, and nervousness. Severe deficiency of B12 causes nerve damage. The *Internet Journal of Nutrition and Wellness* notes that a deficiency of vitamin B12 will quickly reveal its vast importance in the nervous system. For example, a diet insufficient in vitamin B12 can cause central and peripheral nervous system dysfunctions. These can manifest as dementia, muscle spasticity, walking problems, gait abnormalities, weakness, and problems with the bowel and urinary systems.

A neuropathy caused by vitamin B12 deficiency is characterized by numbness in the feet, pins-and-needles sensations, or a burning feeling in the feet. Clinical studies have shown that supplementation of B12 using methylcobalamin to return deficient B12 levels to normal also repairs and restores normal nerve function. This had been used in large part for successful treatment of diabetic neuropathy. In a review of clinical trials conducted between 1954 and 2004, vitamin B12 was shown to reduce pain. Methylcobalamin appears to be the most effective form of vitamin B12 at protecting the nerves.

Vitamin B12 is found naturally in foods such as beef liver, meat, venison, lamb loin, poultry, and seafood such as lobster, clams, oysters, mussels, octopus, salmon, sardines, snapper, and halibut. Other good sources for B vitamins include kombucha, whole (unprocessed) grains, sweet potatoes, bananas, lentils, chili peppers, tempeh, beans, nutritional yeast, brewer's yeast, and molasses, according to *World's Healthiest Foods*, a nonprofit foundation established to share scientifically proven information about the health benefits of eating "whole foods."

All of you beer drinkers, who are thinking you can get a healthy dosage of B12 from your favorite brew, don't rejoice just yet. Although the yeast used to make beer results in it being a source of B vitamins, their bioavailability ranges from poor to none. Drinking ethanol (grain alcohol) inhibits the absorption of thiamine (B_1), riboflavin (B_2), niacin (B_3), biotin (B_7), and folic acid (B_9). There are a vast number of studies that emphasize that elevated consumption of beer and other alcohol-based drinks results in a net deficit of B vitamins, period.

It is uncommon for children and healthy young adults to be deficient in vitamin B12, unless they are vegetarian or vegan, but it's not uncommon for older people to be mildly deficient. As we age, our digestive system loses efficiency in absorbing B-vitamins from the food that we eat. This is often due to the fact that there is less stomach acid production. A person taking certain medications, such as antacids or a group of medications called proton pump inhibitors—like Nexium, Aciphex, Prevacid, or Prilosec—will also encounter malabsorption problems with vitamins. The body is dependent on a healthy supply of hydrochloric acid in the stomach to absorb B12.

Others at risk for B12 deficiency include:

- people with malabsorption disorders (problems absorbing nutrients) due to conditions such as Crohn's disease,

diverticulitis, colitis, and pancreatic disease, and people who have had weight loss surgery;
- people who are infected with *Helicobacter pylori*, an organism in the intestines that can cause an ulcer are at risk for B12 deficiency. H. pylori damages stomach cells that make intrinsic factor, a substance the body needs to absorb B12;
- people with an eating disorder, such as anorexia or bulimia;
- people with HIV;
- the elderly.

Regardless of how healthy you might eat, it's imperative for everyone to take a B-complex supplement daily. For example, my husband and I eat a macrobiotic diet (although we have recently stopped consuming seafood due to the atrocities to our marine wildlife from the fishing industries). We work out four to five days per week. We *never* consume fast food. We drink 2.5–3 liters of purified water daily. We detox twice per year. We're in bed by 9 PM from Sunday through Thursday. We do, however, live wildly on Fridays and Saturdays, going to bed by 10 PM—Woo-hoo!—and sometimes we consume one to two glasses of wine on Fridays and Saturdays, when we're not detoxing. Still, we make sure to take our B-complex daily—among a list of other necessary supplements, such as vitamin D, a whole-food multivitamin, Co-Q10, green tea extract, etc. Why do we do all of this, you ask? B vitamins are water-soluble, and as such they are easily leached out during the cooking process. If you're mostly eating out, I can guarantee that your B-vitamins have been lost in the cooking process before your meal hits the table, even in a five-star restaurant. High-heat cooking (temperatures above 180 degrees) will destroy many vitamins and enzymes in your food. Baking powder is a huge destroyer of B5 (look at your ingredient labels), not to mention that refined grains are deficient in B vitamins. And for you coffee drinkers, every time you urinate after drinking your favorite cup of java, look down into the toilet bowl and wave bye-bye to your B-vitamins (and vitamin C, too). Since coffee acts as a diuretic, all water-soluble vitamins will be washed away.

We've covered a lot of ground, so let's review once more. B vitamins are found in *whole unprocessed foods*. Processed foods such as sugar and white flour have had their B vitamins destroyed in the refining process, resulting in the necessity for enrichment with synthetic B vitamins. Remember, not all B vitamins will be replaced in the process of enrichment. Those that are replaced will still tend to have a lower content of B vitamins than their unprocessed counterparts. We can clearly see that B vitamins are the *heavy hitters* of the nervous system.

9

REBUILDING NERVES...ONE MEAL AT A TIME

"Let food be thy medicine and let medicine be thy food."

Aristotle
(384–322 BC)

You have heard me mention several times throughout this book that vitamin and mineral supplementation is essential, even with a healthy diet; but make no mistake, it still is not a replacement for a sound nutritional diet.

A healthy diet is important for good health in general, but it is especially important for anyone suffering from chronic illnesses, such as peripheral neuropathy. Whole, living foods contain important vitamins, minerals, and coenzymes that promote healing within the body. You might have heard the word *coenzyme* in the past without fully understanding its meaning. A coenzyme is a substance that enhances the action of an enzyme. Your next question is probably, "So, what's an enzyme?" An enzyme is a protein that causes or accelerates a chemical reaction within your body without causing any change to the enzyme itself.

Coenzymes are small, non-protein, organic molecules that enhance the reaction of the enzyme by loosely binding to it. In doing this, the coenzyme helps and supports the function of the enzyme. Because of this, coenzymes play a significant role in the functions of cells. Reactions within the cells either break down nutrients or combine molecules for cellular activities that keep the cells alive. Enzymes speed up these reactions. Without coenzymes, these reactions might not occur.

This is where the problem begins with processed food. The manufacturer would have you believe that you can take a frozen, microwaveable dinner and add in extra vitamins and it will be as nutritious as if you cooked it yourself. They would also have you believe that after the process of pasteurization or refining, which strips away important vitamins, minerals, and nutrients, they can simply add the vitamins back in and everything will be just fine.

As I discussed in the previous chapter, it is rare for the manufacturer to add back in every single nutrient that is lost in the process of refining or pasteurizing food. They also neglect to tell you that while vitamins and minerals can be added to a processed food, coenzyme factors cannot be added back in. What does this mean for your nutrition? Your body will not have the capacity to use the vitamins or minerals the way that they are designed to be used in the cells. Remember, the coenzyme factor is what allows the vitamins and minerals to be absorbed and utilized by the cells. So, whenever you are eating a processed food, you are eating what is known as a dead food.

Let's familiarize ourselves with the concept of "Living Foods" versus "Dead foods"

Living foods are fresh, whole foods that have not been processed, such as fruits, vegetables, nuts, seeds, legumes, and grains. These foods are nutrient-rich and they have the highest density of proteins and phytochemicals. In short, they pack a wallop of health benefits for the body. Dead foods are processed, chemical-laden foods that are devoid of complete nutritional value. When you read the labels on a package of dead foods, you will see ingredients that you typically do not recognize, let alone are able to pronounce.

I have a standard rule of thumb: If you cannot pronounce an ingredient on a label nor identify it as a healthy, whole food source, *don't put it in your mouth!*" Doesn't this sound simple? Due to the processing methods and chemical/preservative additives, dead foods typically *suck* stored vitamins out of your body as your system tries to metabolize them.

All raw foods, of course, are living foods, but a large debate enters in as to whether or not cooked food is living or dead. If you speak to someone who is a raw food purist, they would emphatically say that, without a doubt, all cooked food is dead food. Even though we do agree with the science and philosophy behind the methodology, neither my husband nor I is a raw foodist. The plain truth is that it is a very difficult lifestyle to sustain. When you cook food on high heat, whether it's boiling, frying or baking, you denature or change the chemical composition of the food. Once cooked—or overcooked, we should say—the food can lose up to 85 percent of its original nutritional value, not to mention forming carcinogenic free radicals and advanced glycation end products (AGEs), which are toxins, in the process. At this point, there is no doubt that your food is dead.

Now, for those of you who would rather *die* than go raw—and that's the vast majority of you—you can have your proverbial cake and eat it, too. How do you accomplish this? You should cook using only low heat.

Low heat cooking is a wonderful way to maintain your nutrient content in food. When cooking on a gas range, you should not cook using anything higher than a medium flame. I typically stick with a medium to low flame. If you are using an electric stove, do not set your stovetop settings above the number three. I usually recommend warming your pot or pan at level three and then when the cooktop is preheated, turn the temperature down to two. This will go a long ways toward preserving your nutrients. Slow cookers are also great. When cooking vegetables, resort to steaming and not boiling. Make sure to keep a lid on, which also helps keep nutrients in. Do not steam your vegetables until they are limp and lifeless. Make sure you keep them al dente. They should have a bit of a crunch to them. When I bake in the oven, I do not use temperatures exceeding two hundred degrees. Yes, it takes longer but at least I'm saving my nutrients. The answer to the question I am often asked, "Is it safe to eat chicken cooked at low temperatures?" The answer is a resounding *yes*. Throughout the years, a misconception has formed about food safety and high temperature cooking. We have been taught in order to kill bacteria in food it is necessary to cook meats at 325 degrees or higher. This, however, is not accurate. According to the USDA's guide- listing safe temperatures to reduce salmonella in chicken- the minimum safe cooking temperature for chicken is 165 degrees. The USDA has determined your chicken should be cooked at this temperature for a minimum of 80 minutes in order to accomplish sterilization. Many times, I will do what Mom used to do at Thanksgiving—put the turkey (or chicken) in the oven before going to bed so that it will be ready early the next morning. Don't worry about the length of time your oven is occupied. If you are like the average American, your oven probably has been taken over by cobwebs anyway.

Living foods are typically easier to recognize, but many people are often confused about what are considered dead foods. Here is a list to help you wade through.

LIVING FOOD	DEAD FOOD
1. fruits, fresh;	1. processed food and Junk food;
2. vegetables, fresh;	2. crackers *(all types)*;
3. whole grains;	3. beef jerky *(any type of jerky)*;
4. beans;	4. fruit rollups;
5. nuts and seeds, raw;	5. vegetable chips *(any chip)*;
6. freshly made juices (juicing);	6. boxed cereals *(all brands)*;
7. meat, poultry, fish;	7. bottled fruit juices;
8. sprouted grain bread (e.g., Ezekiel).	8. bread.

The Mayo Clinic recommends a diet that is rich in nutritious fruits and vegetables for those who experience neuropathy.

A healthy diet should include the following types of food:

- Whole grains and beans to provide **B vitamins** in order to promote nerve health. Whole grains promote the production of serotonin in the brain and they will increase your feeling of wellbeing.
- Fish and eggs give you additional **vitamins B12 and B1**.
- Green, leafy vegetables (spinach, kale, and other greens) for **calcium** and **magnesium**. Both of these nutrients are vital for healthy nerve endings and healthy nerve impulse transmission. As an added bonus, they give your immune system a boost.

- Cruciferous vegetables like broccoli, cauliflower, and brussels sprouts are rich in vitamin E.
- Yellow, red, and orange fruits and vegetables (such as sweet potatoes, squash, carrots, yellow, red and orange bell peppers, apricots, oranges, tomatoes, etc.) are rich in **vitamins A and C**, helping repair your skin and boost your immune system.
- Raw and unsalted seeds and nuts, such as sunflower seeds, almonds, hazelnuts, pine nuts, pecans, and Brazil nuts.
- Avocados, sweet potatoes, and fish are rich in **vitamins A, B, C, E**, and minerals like calcium and magnesium.

The Fire Within

Chronic inflammation has been proven to be a common denominator in a whole host of diseases and illnesses, such as cancer, diabetes, depression, heart disease, stroke, Alzheimer's, and even peripheral neuropathy. Inflammation is a normal reaction that occurs in the body and is part of a healthy immune response. Acute inflammation is responsible for breaking down damaged tissue as a way of healing injuries and fighting infections. However, there is an insidious side to inflammation. Chronic hidden inflammation occurs throughout the body when something jump-starts the immune system while simultaneously disengaging the shut-off button that stops inflammation. An untended slow-burning fire then begins, and it will spread. This eventually will lead to a five-alarm fire that burns out of control. What ignites the fires differs from person to person. It can be caused by a variety of factors, including repeated or prolonged infections, smoking, unrelenting levels of stress, and toxic or dead food. Obesity is directly linked to developing chronic inflammation.

Chronic inflammation, whether it is low-level or a full-out raging blaze, is a huge problem with neuropathy sufferers. It is the gasoline that is added to the fire. It causes damage to nerves, blood vessel linings, and many other tissues. In some cases, the chronic ongoing inflammation is what damaged your nerves in the first place; in other cases, it may have not been the cause, but it sure as heck is keeping the fire going. Did you know that being as little as five pounds overweight will start the inflammatory cycle? The more excess body weight you carry, the higher the levels of inflammation within your body. Even sustained levels of chronic stress can cause inflammation to set in and spiral out of control. Other factors contributing to chronic inflammation are a toxic diet, environmental toxins, a lack of movement, a lack of sleep, and GI dysfunction (acid reflux, ulcers, GERD, IBS, etc.) To help protect yourself against all of these factors, it is important to load up on these inflammation-fighting foods. All of the foods that I have listed here have been shown in research to have significant anti-inflammatory properties. This is extremely important when battling peripheral neuropathy.

INFLAMMATION FIGHTING FOODS

(asterisks denote part of the 'dirty dozen')

1. Kelp

Kelp, one of many sea vegetables– such as kombu, contains fucoidan, a type of complex carbohydrate that is anti-inflammatory, antitumor, and antioxidative. This sea vegetable is extremely high in mineral content, especially iodine. Kelp also contains significant levels of beta-carotene, and vitamins B, C, D, E, and K. The high fiber content of kelp also helps induce fullness, slow fat absorption, and promote weight loss. Whenever possible, though, you should get organic kelp that is harvested from the unpolluted sea. Kelp or any sea vegetable is very easy to use; simply add it to your soup or stew, put it in a pot of rice while it is cooking, and presto—you have a mineral-rich food.

2. Wild Alaskan Salmon

Salmon is an excellent source of EPA and DHA, two potent omega-3 fatty acids that douse inflammation. The benefits of omega-3 have been backed by numerous studies, and they range from preventing heart disease and some cancers to reducing the symptoms of autoimmune diseases and psychological disorders. Be sure to include some oily fish, such as wild Alaskan salmon, in your diet twice a week. If you don't enjoy eating fish, you can also get omega-3 fatty acids from high-quality fish oil supplements.

3. Turmeric

This bright orange Asian root spice, which is commonly found in premixed curry powder, contains a powerful, nontoxic compound called curcumin. Studies have found that turmeric's anti-inflammatory effects are on a par with potent drugs, such as hydrocortisone and Motrin. However, it has none of their side effects. Tumeric aids in wound healing, and it helps prevent the progression of inflammatory diseases.

4. Shiitake Mushroom*

Enjoyed by the Chinese and the Japanese since ancient times, shiitake mushrooms are revered for their immune-boosting properties and their mild, smoky taste. The medicinal use of these mushrooms dates back to around 100 AD in China. Research involving the medicinal properties of these gems has been ongoing since the 1960s. Shitake mushrooms are rich in iron, which improves the circulation of oxygen through your blood.

5. Celery*

The polyacetylene in celery provides great relief for all inflammation. A study published in the *Proceedings of the National Academy of Science US.* highlighted the phytonutrient, luteolin, which is found in celery, as inhibiting a pathway that allows for inflammation to set in.

6. Green Tea*

The flavonoids in green tea are potent natural anti-inflammatory compounds that have been shown in numerous studies to reduce the risk of heart disease and cancer. Current research in the January 2011 issue of the *Journal of Food Biochemistry* reported that a strong antioxidant, sunphenon, destroys the free radicals that lead to inflammation. Adding milk to your tea will negate the anti-inflammatory properties. You should only consume organic green tea. Conventionally farmed tealeaves are highly sprayed with pesticides, herbicides, and fungicides. These chemicals increase inflammation and they are neurotoxic.

7. Papaya

Papaya contains papain, a protein-digesting enzyme. Christopher Columbus called this fruit the "fruit of angels." Combined with other nutrients such as vitamins A, C, and E, papain helps reduce inflammation, and it improves immunity and digestion. Dried papaya can be laden with preservatives, which can cause them to lose their anti-inflammatory benefits.

8. Pineapple

Pineapple contains a naturally occurring digestive enzyme called bromelain, which helps break down proteins and aids in digestion. It also reduces swelling and inflammation, and it improves blood circulation. Pineapple is also rich in vitamin C and manganese.

9. Cherries*

The University of Michigan's Cardioprotection Research Laboratory has reported that cherries have the capacity to reduce inflammation around blood vessels. This fruit is high in antioxidants, fiber, and minerals. Cherries contain substantial amounts of vitamin C and beta-carotene, and moderate amounts of vitamin K, vitamin B6, and vitamin A. Some of the minerals found in cherries are potassium, copper, manganese, magnesium, iron, calcium, phosphorus, and zinc. The Linus Pauling Institute at Oregon State University reports that cherries are high in phytosterols, which lower LDL cholesterol and aid in fighting cancer.

10. Ginger

A review published in the *Journal of Medicinal Food* found that ginger's anti-inflammatory properties are comparable to over-the-counter NSAIDs like Advil, Motrin, Aleve, and aspirin without any of the harmful side effects. Aromatic ginger has been touted as a superstar of Asian medicine, according to a review published in the *Journal of Medicinal Food*. It has been treasured for thousands of years for its impressive health benefits. This amazing spice root contains phytonutrients known as gingerols, which are some of the most potent inflammation-fighting substances identified. Ginger extract inhibit several genes that contribute to the formation of inflammation within the body.

11. Garlic

This wonderful herb is power-packed with medicinal benefits. Garlic has been found to lower cholesterol and improve heart health. It also has the ability to stimulate the lymphatic system, which aids in eliminating toxins and reducing whole-body inflammation.

12. Blueberries*

Blueberries are antioxidant powerhouses. They are high in phytonutrients, which provide anti-inflammatory protection against many diseases, such as cancer and dementia. They have enormous benefits in terms of decreasing inflammation within the brain and the nervous system.

13. Broccoli

Broccoli is a highly nutritious vegetable that contains anti-inflammatory and anticancer phytonutrients, such as sulforaphane, which helps the body get rid of potentially carcinogenic compounds. It provides an excellent source of vitamins C and K. Other cruciferous vegetables, such as cauliflower, brussels sprouts, arugula, cabbage, watercress, and chard also contain similar anti-inflammatory and detoxification properties.

14. Spinach*

Spinach is a nutrient-rich vegetable with significant amounts of vitamins K and A, and manganese, folate, magnesium, iron, and much more. Spinach also contains alpha linoleic acid (ALA), which is a form of omega-3 fatty acids that reduce inflammation.

15. Sweet Potatoes*

Sweet potatoes are a great source of beta-carotene, manganese, vitamins B2, B6, C, E, and K, and calcium, folate, iron, magnesium, potassium, and dietary fiber. Together, these nutrients are powerful antioxidants that help heal inflammation in the body. Make sure you buy organic sweet potatoes whenever possible, as they are also among the foods on which pesticide residues have been found the most frequently.

16. Extra Virgin Olive Oil

Virgin olive oil is the Mediterranean secret to longevity. Its rich supply of polyphenols protects the heart and blood vessels from inflammation. Extra virgin olive oil (EVOO) is one of the purest forms of olive oil. In EVOO, no chemicals or heat are used in the oil extraction process. One of the wonderful properties of this oil is that its components are turned into anti-inflammatory agents by the body. This can lower occurrences of asthma, rheumatoid arthritis, and systemic inflammation. Olive oil has a lower smoke point than many other oils, so it should never be used on any heat higher than a medium setting. Otherwise the oil will break down and form dangerous free radicals in the cooking process. Once this occurs, all of the health benefits are tossed out the window.

17. Coconut Oil

Virgin coconut oil helps treat chronic inflammation, as reported in a study published in the February 2010 issue of *Pharmaceutical Biology*. As published in *Medical Principles and Practice* in March 2011, virgin coconut oil, which is high in lauric acid, caprylic acid, and capric acid, is tremendously effective in reducing inflammation and aiding in the treatment of conditions like heart disease, high blood pressure, diabetes, and certain cancers. Always use unrefined (or virgin) cold-pressed coconut oil. It also makes a wonderful skin moisturizer for your body.

18. Ghee

Ghee has been used for over two thousand years in India as part of their Ayurvedic medicine system, which is an ancient natural healing system. Ghee is clarified butter with the milk protein removed, leaving rich, and delicious pure butter fat. This oil is free of casein, the culprit in asthma and dairy sensitivities, making it safe for lactose-intolerant people. Lab studies have shown that ghee reduces cholesterol, improves gallbladder function, and promotes nerve and brain health. This oil has been found to promote learning and increase memory retention. Ghee is rich in antioxidants, which squelch free radicals and aid in decreasing inflammation. It contains a high concentration of butyric acid, which has antiviral properties and antitumor properties. It also contains conjugated linoleic acid (CLA), which aids in weight loss. Ghee is high in vitamins A, D, E, and K.

Note: The following oils should never be used for cooking, due to their low smoke points and/or genetic modification: flaxseed, safflower, sunflower, soy, peanut, corn oils.

Menu Planning:

Several times throughout this book, we've mentioned the importance of improving the way you eat. Notice that we did not use the term *diet*. I have never liked this term. Webster's dictionary defines the word *diet* as "a food and drink that is regularly consumed by a person or animal." However, over time we have come to identify the word *diet* with stringent regulations and restrictions on food intake for the purposes of weight loss.

One's goal should never be dieting, even when your objective is weight loss. After all, look at the first three letters of the word: D-I-E. Don't you think that says it all? Dieting rarely works. Sure, you might lose significant amounts of weight, but statistics show that more than 80 percent of people who have lost weight regain all of it, or more, after two years. Researchers at the University of California at Los Angeles analyzed thirty-one long-term diet studies, and they found that approximately two-thirds of dieters regained more weight within four or five years than they initially lost. Whether your goal is weight loss or, in this case, regaining your health, you should never diet.

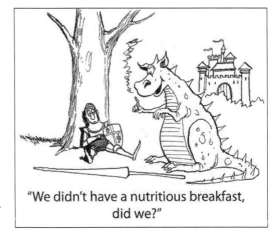

"We didn't have a nutritious breakfast, did we?"

What you should do is embark on a ***therapeutic lifestyle change*** program. How do these two approaches differ? When dieting, you remove all of the bad food that you have been eating, and you drastically reduce your calories until you lose the weight. Most often this leaves you hungry, unsatisfied, and feeling deprived. Once the weight is lost, you end up reverting to your old eating habits, which results in regaining most, if not all or more, of the weight you had initially lost. This is very different from a therapeutic lifestyle change (TLC). A therapeutic lifestyle change (TLC) means that you live your life and make choices daily that improve your health. As reported by the National Institutes of Health, using a TLC approach is far more effective for losing weight, achieving great health, and preventing many illnesses. Anyone can achieve a TLC by being educated about which choices truly are healthful for you. Unfortunately, most people rely on the deceptive world of advertising to teach them about what is healthy. If this is your only base of knowledge, you will likely be led astray, repeatedly.

Utilizing the TLC approach will enable you to prevent illness and aid in healing. Even more exciting, it will allow you to live your life to the fullest, waking up and feeling good every day. Unlike a diet, a TLC program does not leave you hungry. It's not about being on severe caloric restriction or being on a vegetarian diet. As a matter of fact, you will be able to eat more than you ever thought possible without gaining weight. Let's keep it real. If your taste buds have been acclimated to loads of sugar and processed foods for your entire life, will it take some adjusting? Yes it will. But I promise you that the adjustments are much easier than you would ever anticipate. Most important, later on in this chapter, I will provide you with healthy recipes that are absolutely delicious!

Lies we tell ourselves…

We have convinced ourselves that food is merely an energy source for the body; therefore, all food is created equal. In the back of our mind, we realize that there is no way, from a nutritional standpoint, that a candy bar can compare to a bowl of fruit. However, we lull ourselves into a false sense of security, because after all food is just fuel. In reality, the food that you eat supplies much more for your body than just energy or fuel. It provides the raw materials from which your nerves, muscles, bones, organs, and all of your other tissues are made. Whole, living food is also necessary for manufacturing hormones and enzymes, and for repairing all of the tissues in the body when they are damaged. Your candy bar or bag of chips may indeed provide you with fuel—albeit, the poorest-quality fuel—but it cannot provide the foundation for cellular repair. Here are some basics that you will need to know to start making better choices for your health.

Good Health and the Sugar Connection

We mentioned earlier that chronic inflammation is capable of doing extensive damage to nerves over time. One of the biggest culprits leading to chronic inflammation is the spikes in your blood sugar levels (glucose). Chronic spikes in blood glucose will eventually lead to insulin resistance. This doesn't necessarily mean that you have diabetes. However if this continues, eventually it's not a matter of *if* you will develop diabetes—it's a matter of *when* you will develop diabetes.

When making good food choices, it is important to choose foods with a low glycemic index. Through the process of digestion, food gets broken down into small molecules that can be absorbed in your bloodstream and utilized by your cells for energy. Low glycemic index means that the food produces a low level of blood sugar when it is broken down. Conversely, a food with a high glycemic index will produce high levels of sugar, which gets dumped into the bloodstream very rapidly. There is a direct correlation to chronic spikes in blood sugar and inflammation.

Understanding Fat, Protein, and Carbohydrates

Carbohydrates

Carbohydrates have been given a bad rap over the past few years, especially with the introduction of the Atkins diet. Whole-food carbohydrates, such as sweet potatoes, are a good source of energy, fiber, vitamins, and minerals. Whole-food carbohydrates that have a moderate-to-high fiber content do not have a high glycemic index, unlike white potatoes. Consuming whole-food, high-fiber carbohydrates is not problematic for your health or weight loss; consuming processed, refined carbohydrates with little to no fiber creates a health burden. An example would be a diet loaded with bread made from refined flour (white or wheat), crackers, cookies, chips, French fries, etc. These refined carbohydrates result in a high glycemic index with sharp glucose spikes, or in simpler terms—a large and fast *sugar dump into the bloodstream.* This leads to high levels of inflammation. You should strive to get your carbohydrates from whole foods, such as high fiber fruits, vegetables, beans, lentils, and whole grains.

Fat

For years, many people believed that low-fat meant good health. If this were true, with all of the low-fat, processed food on the grocery store shelves, we should have a thin society. However, Americans are fatter than ever. It is not only good for you to eat fat from whole-food sources in moderation; it is necessary. We need fat to make hormones and for other physiological functions.

The problem with processed foods that are labeled "low fat" is the added sugar content. Once the manufacturer has removed the fat, they must add in greater amounts of refined sugar to give the product its taste appeal. This leads to spikes in blood glucose and increases of insulin secretion. Your body can actually turn excess sugar into fat.

The good news about the right type of fats is that it actually slows the rate that sugar gets dumped into the bloodstream. Remember, even good fat should be eaten with moderation. It should not make up more than 20–30 percent of your percent of your caloric intake.

Good Fats	Bad Fats
<ul><li>Avocados</li><li>Cold water fish</li><li>Raw nuts/nut butters (not peanuts)</li><li>Raw seeds</li><li>Fish oil/krill oil</li><li>Olive oil (extra virgin)</li><li>Flaxseed oil</li><li>Coconut oil</li><li>Ghee</li><li>Sesame Oil</li></ul>	<ul><li>Junk food/snacks</li><li>Crackers</li><li>Whole fat, pasteurized dairy products (milk, cream, ice cream)</li><li>Margarine</li><li>Shortening/lard</li><li>Fried foods</li><li>Candy bars</li></ul>

Protein

Protein is a necessary component for making muscle, skin, and hair, as well as other tissues. It is also necessary to manufacture necessary hormones and enzymes that are involved in tissue repair and regeneration, metabolism, and digestion. Red meat is no longer the villain it was once made out to be. In a 2010 study published in the *American Journal of Clinical Nutrition*, it was found that increased intakes of saturated fat did not lead to increased cholesterol or heart disease. What was shown to have a direct link to these diseases were high carbohydrate diets, that is, refined carbohydrates. Large intakes of refined carbohydrates increased insulin resistance, which leads to glucose spikes, fat deposition, and inflammation. It's time to celebrate! No longer do you have to fear eating red meat. What is important is the type of red meat that you eat. Conventionally raised, grain-fed red meat increases the inflammatory cascade. Conventional red meat is laden with hormones and antibiotics. It is also lower in omega-3 fatty acids. Grass-fed red meat is very high in omega-3s. Whenever you eat red meat, always opt for organic, grass-fed red meat. This is the healthiest form of red meat.

Chicken, which was once thought to be the health-food hero, has actually been linked to causing inflammation. Turkey, although still part of the poultry family, has not been found to elicit an inflammatory cascade. The same principles apply to chicken as beef. You should always purchase organic, free-range chicken.

Both red meat and poultry consumption should be limited to only two to three times per week. Cold-water fish is an excellent source of omega-3 fatty acids. Make sure to check the list in chapter 5 for the mercury content in fish.

Fiber

Dietary fiber plays a significant role in promoting healthy insulin and sugar response. Diets that are high in fiber prevent a fast surge of glucose– eliminating spikes that lead to chronic inflammation. Good sources of fiber include apples, cherries, prunes, beans, brown rice, raw nuts, green vegetables (the crunchier, the better), and whole grains like oats, quinoa, and millet.

Water

Water intake and fluid balance are the least understood areas of health. Your life and health are fully dependent upon water for proper function. The human body is comprised of approximately 70 percent water. There are an estimated one hundred trillion cells in the human body. When the body lacks sufficient water, these cells begin to desiccate (dry up), causing their inner processes to malfunction. This is a precipitating factor in chronic inflammation.

It's estimated that **about 75 percent of Americans are chronically dehydrated.** Many of you have heard that each day, you should be consuming half of your body weight in ounces of water. For instance, a two-hundred-pound individual should consume approximately one hundred ounces of water (or three liters). Most of you have dropped to the floor just now because you probably barely consume sixteen ounces (two glasses) of water per day. You don't like the taste of water? That is the lamest excuse in the book. I don't know very many people who enjoyed the taste of alcohol—-whether it was beer, wine, rum, vodka, or whiskey—the first time they had a drink. And how about that first cigarette that you choked on? Oh yes, that was a real treat, wasn't it? My point is that you can acquire a taste for anything if you make an attempt. Try squeezing some fresh lemons or limes into your water to help you acquire a taste. Once you do this, nothing else will ever quench your thirst again.

Tea, coffee, juice, alcohol, and sodas *cannot be substituted for water.* Fluids that contain caffeine and alcohol have a diuretic effect, causing the kidneys to flush some of the body's water reserves.

Here is a strategy for helping you increase your fluid intake. As soon as you get out of bed in the morning, consume eight ounces of water right off the bat. This will help with hydration, and it will help your energy and mental clarity. Next, take any one-liter bottle (thirty-three ounces) and fill it up (*do not use tap water*). Carry this bottle around with you and sip constantly throughout the day. Do not refill this bottle until it is empty. Your goal is to reach a bare minimum consumption of two liters of water per day.

Here is a sample list of foods that will help you decrease inflammation and toxic loads in your body:

CATEGORIES	INCLUDE - THESE FOODS	EXCLUDE - THESE FOODS
Fruits	Unsweetened fresh, frozen, or bottled fruit juices (preferably organic)	*No* orange juice *No* oranges
Vegetables	All fresh, raw, steamed, sautéed, juiced, or roasted vegetables	*No* corn, canned, or creamed vegetables
Grains	Brown rice (short or long grain), wild rice, millet, oats, teff, quinoa, amaranth, buckwheat	*No* white rice, wheat, corn, barley, spelt, kamut, rye; any grains with gluten

CATEGORIES	INCLUDE - THESE FOODS	EXCLUDE - THESE FOODS
Bread / Cereal Ezekiel sprouted grain, Food for Life-millet, Exotic black rice	Products made from rice, oat, buckwheat, millet, quinoa, teff, amaranth, tapioca, arrowroot, potato flour, rice crackers	*No* products with wheat, spelt, kamut, rye, barley; any gluten containing grain.
Legumes / Beans	All beans, peas and lentils (soak all raw beans for 48 hours and change water)	*No* soybeans, tofu, tempeh, soy milk, or other soy products (except organic tamari)
Nuts and Seeds Raw Only	Almonds, cashews, walnuts, pecans, sesame, tahini, sunflower, pumpkin seeds or any nut butters made from these nuts	*No* peanuts or peanut butter
Meat and Fish	Frozen or fresh fish, chicken, turkey, wild game, lamb, Applegate Farms organic sliced turkey sandwich meat, and organic turkey-bacon, organic cage free eggs.	*No* beef, pork, hot dogs, sausage, bacon, canned meats, shellfish, no cold cuts/sandwich meats not specified
Dairy Products and Milk Substitutes	Unsweetened: rice milk, almond milk, coconut milk (SO*), oat milk, hazelnut milk, other unsweetened nut milks	*No* milk, cheese, cottage cheese, yogurt, cream/half and half, butter, ice cream, nondairy creamers
Fats	Ghee, extra-virgin olive oil, coconut oil walnut oil, pumpkin oil, almond oil, flaxseed oil (do not heat flax oil)	*No* butter, margarine, shortening, vegetable oils, hydrogenated oils, mayonnaise
Beverages	Spring, filtered, or sparkling water, Teecino (coffee sub) herbal or green teas you may have iced tea made from herbal teas.	*No* soda or soft drinks, alcohol, coffee, black tea, sweet tea, regular iced tea

CATEGORIES	INCLUDE - THESE FOODS	EXCLUDE - THESE FOODS
Spices, Herbs, and Condiments SO Herbs, Frontier	Any fresh or dried organic spice-herb (unless otherwise indicated), Bragg's Liquid Aminos, organic tamari sauce Celtic sea salt, Mediterranean pink sea salt, whole grain organic mustard, Muir Glen organic ketchup,	*No* chocolate, soy sauce, ketchup, mustard, relish, BBQ sauce or other condiments not specified
Sweeteners	Sweet Leaf Stevia, Xylo-Sweet, Xyla (by Emerald Forest), brown rice syrup, raw honey, blackstrap molasses	*No* white or brown sugar, maple syrup, corn syrup, high fructose corn syrup, Truvia, Splenda, Equal, Nutrasweet, Sweet'n Low, candy, desserts

Note: do not confuse coconut milk with coconut cream. Coconut milk has the same consistency as soy milk. Make sure all nut milks are unsweetened.

JUICING

With leading organizations like the National Institutes of Health and the National Cancer Society stating that we need to incorporate at least five servings of fruits and vegetables into our daily intake, more people are discovering the benefits of juicing. In the latest research findings, children and adults were reported to be consuming only one cup of vegetables per day and less than half a cup of fruit—abysmal statistics. It can be daunting for the average person to consume the recommended daily amounts of fruits and vegetables. Juicing makes it easy to meet these requirements.

While you can certainly juice fruits, if you suffer from diabetes, prediabetes, elevated cholesterol or high blood pressure, it is best to limit these juices. Raw fruit juice is high in fructose (natural fruit sugar), which tends to increase glucose and insulin levels in the body. Vegetable juicing, on the other hand, is critical to good health. Green juices (juice primarily made by green vegetables) are an important source of raw food and are an excellent way to deliver high-quality nutrition to the cells of your body, thereby aiding in the recovery process. When you drink live juices, your cells are flooded with the nutrients that are necessary for rebuilding your tissues and repairing any damage. Some of the most important ingredients from raw juices are the active enzymes that your body uses to transform nutrients into a usable form for cellular growth and overall health. Commercial bottled juices that you find in a store have been pasteurized, thereby killing off the active enzymes.

Did you know in the juiced form, nutrients are very easy to assimilate? Typically, most patients who suffer from peripheral neuropathy, chronic inflammation, and other degenerative types of illness have difficulty digesting food properly. Bloating after meals, burping, gas, cramping, heartburn, or acid reflux are a few of the many indications that you might have poor digestion. Many medications can also cause a dysfunctional digestive tract. Since raw juice is packed with enzymes, very little effort is required by your digestive tract to assimilate the nutrients into your cells.

Recommendations for Juicing:

1. **Don't juice beets alone.** Beets are a potent detoxifier of the liver, which can overwhelm a feeble person's system. When juicing, you should combine beets with other veg-

etables, like greens, cucumbers, and celery. Don't skip the beets, though; they have amazing health benefits. They are high in potassium, phosphorous, calcium, magnesium, folate, and fiber. Beets also have a good supply of niacin, vitamin C, and vitamin A. *(Note: Juicing or eating beets can turn your feces or urine red. Don't be alarmed. It's not blood– it's the natural food color of the beets.)*

2. **Fresher is better**. Raw juice contains its highest amount of nutrients soon after juicing. When the juice comes in contact with oxygen, it begins to oxidize, losing valuable nutrients. Make sure to store any juice not consumed in a glass, airtight container.

3. **Go Organic**. Conventional produce is laden with pesticides, herbicides, and fungicides. Simply washing or soaking your produce will only eliminate what is on the surface. Many chemicals will still be present in the flesh of the produce. If you can't afford to do all organic juicing, at least use organic produce for the dirty dozen–produce with the highest concentration of pesticides. *(download the dirty dozen app to your smart phone or visit: http://www.ewg.org/foodnews/ for a complete list).*

4. **Save the Pulp.** Don't throw the leftover pulp away. It's a great source of fiber. Stir it into soups or stews. Use in place of breadcrumbs when making something like meatballs or meatloaf. Use it in a baking recipe for healthy muffins or in pancakes to increase your fiber content. Throw some pulp into your breakfast smoothies.

5. **Less is Better.** Don't go crazy mixing together too many vegetables. It can sometimes distort the taste of your juice.

Juicing Recipes To Jumpstart Your Health:

Red Punch (Dr. M's Favorite): *This juice is great for the liver, colon, and digestive tract.*

- 3–4 carrots
- 1 celery stalk *(optional—celery is a great diuretic)*
- 1/4 beet
- 1 apple
- 1/2 oz. ginger *(This is optional.* **Ginger is great for nerve pain,** *and it decreases chronic inflammation, lowering the inflammation of all of the nerves in your body. Ginger makes your drink spicy, however.)*

Green Lemonade (Dr. C's favorite): *Green juicing is very important. It will stop the cycle of chronic inflammation. Juicing cucumbers, celery, kale, parsley, spinach, broccoli, and any other greens will get you back on track.*

- 3 red apples
- 1 lime (remove seeds but keep skin on)
- 2 lemons (remove seeds and skin)
- 3-inch piece, fresh-peeled ginger
- 3 leaves kale (remove thick stem)
- 1/2 bunch of organic spinach
- 1 small handful Italian leaf parsley (1/2 small bunch)
- 1 small handful cilantro, (1/2 small bunch)
- 1 peeled cucumber (preferably seedless)

NOTE: *When juicing with beets, carrots, and apples, once the fiber is removed from the juice the glycemic index (sugar volume dumped into the bloodstream) becomes high. To slow this down, simply add one tablespoon of inulin fiber to your juice and stir. Inulin is a soluble vegetable fiber. The most common source of this fiber is the chicory plant. It will slow down the rate that the sugar is released into your bloodstream. Metamucil sells a high-quality inulin fiber that is labeled as, "Metamucil—Clear & Natural." It dissolves easily in liquids. I do not recommend using regular Metamucil. Although it is a good source of insoluble fiber, it does not dissolve and will make your juice unpleasantly thick.*

SAMPLE MENU PLAN:

Here are some options for foods that you can put together for a meal plan. Get creative and have fun with it.

Breakfast: A bowl of quinoa with 1 teaspoon of fresh ground flax sprinkled with cinnamon and chopped raw nuts.

Or

2 cage-free, organic eggs, cooked lightly over or sunny-side up, on top of 1/2–1 cup of brown rice, topped with dill and cilantro. Sliced tomatoes on the side.

Snack: 8 ounces of freshly made vegetable juice combo or a serving of fruit.

Lunch: Protein (listed in the 'Foods to Include' table), baked sweet potato or rice, and a large side of vegetables.

Snack: Hummus with celery sticks and rice crackers.

Dinner: Joanna's turkey skillet, spaghetti squash, and large salad.

Recipes to get you started

Learning how to prepare some of these foods, which may be new to you, can be overwhelming. I've included some of our favorite recipes that we share with our patients. Each recipe I have included for you has received rave reviews, even from our die-hard junk food junkies.

Morning Meals:

Apples and Cinnamon Breakfast Quinoa

Ingredients:

- 1 cup dry quinoa, rinsed well
- 1 ½ cups water
- 1 teaspoon cinnamon and more for sprinkling
- 2 teaspoons vanilla extract
- ½ cup unsweetened organic applesauce
- ¼ cup organic golden raisins
- 1 cup warmed unsweetened coconut milk for drizzling (any nut milk is fine)
- 1 organic apple, peeled and diced
- ¼ cup raw pecans, chopped

Directions:

1. Combine quinoa, water, cinnamon, and vanilla in a small saucepan and bring it to a boil.
2. Reduce to a simmer, cover, and let it cook for fifteen minutes, until quinoa can be fluffed with a fork.
3. Stir in the applesauce and raisins, and pour in warmed milk. Divide cooked quinoa into four servings. Top off with freshly cut apples, pecans, and a dash of cinnamon.

Dr. C's Outrageous Oatmeal

Ingredients:

- ½ cup of Arrowhead Mills steel cut oats
- ½ cup filtered water
- 1 teaspoon ground flax meal
- 1 teaspoon real vanilla extract
- 1 teaspoon coconut oil
- 1 teaspoon organic raw honey
- 2 tablespoons berries
- 2 tablespoons protein powder (whey) *(optional)*
- nuts *(optional)*

Directions:

1. Combine water and oats in a saucepan and bring to gentle boil.
2. Reduce the heat to simmer, leave uncovered, and stir frequently.
3. Allow the water to evaporate

4. Remove pan from the heat once the desired consistency is reached (10-15 minutes).
5. Add coconut oil, ground flax, and vanilla extract, and blend (flax will thicken the oatmeal).
6. Serve in a bowl and top with berries.
7. Add honey to sweeten.

Breakfast Burrito

Ingredients:

- 2 eggs
- 2 tablespoons water
- 2 tablespoons green and red bell peppers
- 1 jalapeño pepper *(optional)*
- 2 tablespoons green onions/scallions
- 2 tablespoons mushrooms *(optional)*
- 1 Ezekiel tortilla wrap
- salsa (topping)
- ½ tablespoon ghee
- Celtic sea salt and black pepper *(to taste)*

Directions:

1. In a bowl, add eggs, water, salt, and pepper. Beat with a whisk and set it aside.
2. Preheat the skillet on medium heat with ½ tablespoon of ghee.
3. Add the egg mixture to the pan and mix it with wooden spoon or spatula as it sets.
4. Add in the desired vegetables.

5. Place the egg mixture in a tortilla and roll it.
6. Wrap in wax paper
7. Add salsa right before eating *(to prevent sogginess)*

Rise and Shine Pancakes—*Gluten Free*

Ingredients:

- ¼ cup almond flour plus 2 tablespoons
- ½ cup millet flour
- 2 tablespoons rice flour
- 1 teaspoon guar gum or xanthan gum
- ½ teaspoon celtic salt (fine)
- ½ teaspoon baking soda
- ½ teaspoon baking powder
- 1 teaspoon cinnamon
- 2 large eggs (beaten)
- 1 cup buttermilk (organic)
- 2 tablespoons ghee (melted)

Directions:

1. Preheat the oven to 170° F.
2. In a large bowl, combine the dry ingredients and stir with a whisk to blend (you can keep the blend in an airtight container in a cool, dry place for up to three months).
3. Add the eggs, buttermilk, and melted butter to the dry ingredients and stir just until smooth. Do not overmix it.
4. Heat a large skillet or griddle over medium-low heat. Melt about a teaspoon of ghee or coconut oil. Test that

the surface is hot enough by running your hands under the faucet to wet your fingertips; then shake them over the hot griddle. If the water dances across the pan, the heat is just right to begin making your pancakes.
5. For each large pancake, pour ¼ cup of batter into the pan. Cook until bubbles form on the top of each pancake; flip and cook until golden brown on the bottom.
6. Transfer to a baking sheet and keep warm in the oven while cooking the remaining batter, slicking the skillet with a small amount of ghee or coconut oil occasionally, as needed.

Variations: Try adding fresh fruit, such as ½ cup of blueberries or sliced bananas, and a few dashes of cinnamon. Add the ground cinnamon directly to the batter and whisk to incorporate. Simply sprinkle the fresh fruit on top of each pancake before you flip it over.

Raspberry Honey Sauce

Ingredients:

- 1 cup raw honey
- 1 cup fresh or frozen organic raspberries

Directions:

1. Heat the honey in a small saucepan over low heat until it is liquefied.
2. Add raspberries to the honey. Cook, stirring occasionally, until the berries start falling apart.

3. Serve it in a spouted pitcher.
4. Pour it over pancakes.

Soups

Mexican Fiesta Soup *(spicy)*

Ingredients:

- 1 ½ pounds boneless skinless chicken breasts
- 2 tablespoons olive oil
- 1 large red onion, diced
- 1 jalapeno pepper, diced (seeds included)
- 4 cloves garlic, minced
- 1 poblano pepper, diced
- 2 teaspoons chili powder
- 2 teaspoons cumin
- 2 Calabasa squash (sliced and quartered)
- 1 tablespoon Mexican fiesta seasoning (Frontier)
- 2 teaspoons Celtic sea salt
- 8 cups chicken broth (2 quarts)
- 1 4-ounce can diced green chilies
- 3 cups black beans, soaked and rinsed
- 1-14 ounce can Muir Glen organic fire roasted diced tomatoes
- Juice from 2 limes
- 1 cup chopped cilantro stems
- chopped cilantro leaves for serving

Directions:

1. Heat the olive oil over medium heat in a Dutch oven or very large pot. Once it is hot, add the diced onion and the jalapeno and cook for five minutes, until soft. Add the garlic, cubed chicken, diced poblano pepper. Stir and cook for another two minutes. Add the chili powder, Mexican fiesta seasoning, and cumin. Mix until it is well combined.
2. Pour in the chicken stock. Add the diced tomatoes, black beans, green chilies, chopped cilantro stems. Bring this to a low boil, and then reduce to a simmer for forty-five minutes.
3. Finally, add lime juice. Serve with chopped cilantro on the side

Note: to make this meal vegetarian, simply omit the chicken and use vegetable broth.

Chicken and Rice Soup

Ingredients:

- 2 tablespoons olive oil (EVOO)
- 1 chicken (3 pounds) boned, skinned, and visible fat removed, diced
- 3 quarts chicken stock (organic)
- ¼ cup sea vegetables (kelp, arame, wakame)
- 1 ½ cups chopped onions

- 1 cup chopped celery
- 1 cup diced carrots
- ½ cup chopped green onions
- 4 cloves garlic, minced
- ¼ cup fresh parsley leaves
- 2 tablespoons fresh basil, chopped
- 1 cup fresh green beans (organic), chopped
- 1 cup zucchini, diced
- 1 1/2 cups torn kale leaves, cleaned and stemmed
- 1 whole jalapeno, unseeded *(optional)*
- ½ cup wild rice, uncooked
- 2 tablespoons paprika
- 1 tablespoon oregano
- 1 tablespoon thyme
- 2 tablespoons Celtic sea salt
- 1 tablespoon black pepper

Directions:

1. In a large saucepot, heat the olive oil on medium-low heat. When the oil is hot, add the chicken and the garlic and sauté it for about five minutes, or until the meat is slightly browned.
2. Add the stock, sea vegetables, onions, celery, carrots, kale, green onions, wild rice, and all of the herbs and spices. Bring this to a boil and then immediately turn the heat to low. Simmer for thirty minutes.
3. Add all of the remaining vegetables and simmer for fifteen minutes longer or until the rice and veggies are tender.

Side Dishes

Sesame Kale

Ingredients:

- 3 bunches kale (3 lbs.)
- 1 tablespoon sesame oil
- 3 cloves garlic, chopped or minced
- 2 tablespoons water
- 1 tablespoon tamari sauce, low sodium
- 2 teaspoons sesame seeds
- Celtic sea salt and pepper to taste

Directions:

1. Wash bunches of kale and shake out the excess water.
2. Remove and discard the stems from the kale and tear the kale into pieces.
3. Chop or mince the garlic.
4. Preheat the skillet with sesame oil over medium-low heat.
5. Add the garlic to hot oil and sauté it for twenty seconds.
6. Add the kale and water and stir it frequently until kale is wilted.
7. Stir in the tamari sauce, sesame seeds, and salt and pepper

Asparagus With Roasted Peppers and Olives

Ingredients:

- 1 sweet red pepper
- 1 pound asparagus, cut into 1" pieces

- 1 tablespoon of ghee
- 2 cloves garlic, minced
- 2 tablespoons lemon juice
- 2 tablespoons pitted kalamata olives
- 1 tablespoon chopped fresh Italian parsley
- 1 teaspoon each of Celtic sea salt and black pepper

Serves 4

Directions:

1. In a large skillet over medium heat, melt the ghee.
2. Add the asparagus and garlic and cook for five minutes, stirring constantly.
3. Add the lemon juice, cover, and cook for two minutes, or until the asparagus is bright green, crisp, and tender.
4. Add red peppers and cook for one more minute, stirring frequently.
5. Remove from the heat. Stir in the olives and parsley. Add salt and black pepper to taste.
6. Serve it warm.

Beans and Legumes

Black Beans

Ingredients:

- 1 cup black beans, soaked
- 2 cups broth or water

- 1 small onion, chopped
- 2 clove garlic, chopped
- ¼ cup chopped fresh cilantro *(stems and leaves)*
- ¼ teaspoon cayenne pepper *(optional)*
- 1 teaspoon Celtic sea salt

Directions:

1. In a medium saucepan, combine water, beans, onion, garlic, salt, and cayenne and bring it to a boil.
2. Reduce the heat to low and simmer for thirty to forty-five minutes (until the beans are tender).
3. Season it with cilantro, cayenne, and salt. Simmer for five minutes, and serve.

Zesty Kale and Lentils

Ingredients:

- 2 tablespoons extra virgin olive oil
- 1 large onion, finely chopped
- 1 large garlic clove, crushed
- ½ tablespoon ground cumin
- ½ teaspoon ground ginger
- 1 cup French green or red lentils
- 2½ cups vegetable broth
- 1 bunch kale leaves
- 2 tablespoons of fresh mint leaves
- 1 tablespoon of fresh cilantro
- 1 tablespoon of fresh flat parsley leaves

- 1 whole lime, freshly squeezed
- 1 teaspoon of Celtic sea salt and pepper

Directions:

1. Heat oil in a large skillet over medium heat. Add the onion and cook for six minutes, stirring often.
2. Stir in the garlic, cumin, and ginger. Cook this, stirring occasionally until onion starts to brown.
3. Stir in lentils. Pour in enough broth to cover the lentils and bring it to a boil.
4. Lower the heat to a simmer for twenty to thirty minutes (until it is tender).
5. Rinse the kale leaves in cold water and spin dry. You may chop or slice the leaves.
6. Finely chop the mint, cilantro, and parsley leaves.
7. Add kale to the cooked lentils (if broth has dried up, add a bit more). Stir until it is slightly wilted.
8. Stir in the mint, cilantro, and parsley.
9. Add lime juice, sea salt, and pepper to taste.
10. Mix and serve.

Main Dishes

Vegetarian Curry *(good for fighting inflammation)*

Ingredients:

- 2 tablespoons of ghee
- 1 cup of onion, chopped

- ✥ 3 cloves of garlic, minced
- ✥ 4 teaspoons of fresh ginger, minced
- ✥ 1 cup of crushed tomatoes (fresh or Muir Glen Organic)
- ✥ 3 cups of water
- ✥ 1 teaspoon of turmeric
- ✥ 1 teaspoon of cumin
- ✥ 1 teaspoon of cardamom, ground
- ✥ ½ teaspoon of Celtic sea salt
- ✥ ½ teaspoon of cayenne pepper
- ✥ 8 cups of cauliflower florets
- ✥ 2 cups of cooked garbanzo beans (presoaked)
- ✥ 1 cup of peas
- ✥ ½ cup of parsley, chopped

1. In a large heavy-bottomed pot, heat the oil over medium heat and add onion, garlic, and ginger. Sauté this for about five minutes. Add crushed tomatoes, water, turmeric, cumin, cardamom, salt, and cayenne pepper, stirring to mix.
2. Add the cauliflower, beans, and peas to the sauce mixture. Stir until it is fully coated with the sauce, then cover the pot and simmer for seven to eight minutes, until the cauliflower is tender enough for your fork to pierce it. Add parsley, stirring to combine, and then serve over rice, quinoa, or millet.

Serves four.

Turkey and Cabbage Skillet

Ingredients:

- 1 pound of ground turkey breast
- 1 medium yellow onion, chopped
- 1 green bell pepper
- 1 red bell pepper
- 8 ounces of sliced mushrooms
- 3 tablespoons of Italian seasonings
- 1 can (28 ounce) of Muir Glen organic crushed/diced tomatoes
- 8 cups shredded cabbage (about 1 pound)
- 2 garlic cloves, minced
- 1 teaspoon of fresh thyme leaves, chopped
- 3 tablespoons of chopped, fresh dill
- 1 cup of water
- ½ cup of brown rice, uncooked
- 2 teaspoons of Celtic sea salt

Directions:

1. Brown meat, onion, garlic, thyme, and Italian seasonings in a large skillet or a Dutch oven on medium-high heat for four to six minutes or until the meat is cooked through.
2. Add tomatoes, water, rice, cabbage and salt, and stir it. Reduce the heat to a simmer and cover it tightly. Cook for twenty to twenty-five minutes, or until the cabbage and the rice are tender.
3. Add peppers and mushrooms. Cover tightly and simmer for 10 minutes longer.

4. Remove from heat and let it stand, covered, for five minutes and then serve it.

Rice Gone Nuts

Ingredients:

- 1 cup of short grain brown rice
- 2 cups of organic chicken or vegetable broth
- 1/8 cup sea vegetables (kelp, arame)
- 4 garlic cloves
- ½ cup of carrots, shredded
- 3 teaspoons of Celtic sea salt
- 1 teaspoon of extra virgin olive oil
- 1 small bunch of fresh parsley, minced
- Juice of 2 limes
- ½ cup almonds

Directions:

1. Place bunch of parsley (leaves and stems) in food processor and mince, then set aside
2. Mince the garlic, nuts and juice from the limes in processor.
3. Combine parsley, garlic, nut mixture in a bowl and set aside, once again
4. In a medium pot, add the rice, sea vegetables and salt to the broth, and bring to a boil.
5. Reduce the heat to a simmer, cover the pan with a tight-fitting lid, and cook rice for forty minutes or until dry and fluffy.

6. Mix in the carrot once the rice is cooked. Remove from heat but let it sit, covered, for five minutes.
7. Remove lid and allow rice to cool for 20 minutes
8. Add the parsley, garlic and nut mixture into the rice and stir until nut mixture is equally distributed throughout.
9. Portion and serve.

Mediterranean Rice Salad

Ingredients:

- 1 cup brown basmati rice
- 2 cups water
- 5 tablespoons extra virgin olive oil
- 3 tablespoons lime juice, fresh
- 1 tablespoon fresh oregano
- ½ teaspoon whole grain mustard
- 2 large ripe tomatoes, deseeded and chopped
- 1 red bell pepper, deseeded and chopped
- ¾ cup kalamata olives, pitted and halved
- 1 tablespoon capers, rinsed and drained
- 1 cup fresh Italian leaf parsley, chopped
- 1 ½ teaspoon Celtic sea salt (set aside 1/2 teaspoon)
- 1 teaspoon fresh ground peppercorns
- Diced cucumber (to garnish)

Directions:

1. In a large pan, bring water to a boil with ½ teaspoon of sea salt added.

2. Add the rice and stir. Cover and simmer for thirty to forty-five minutes, until the rice is dry and tender.
3. Whisk the extra virgin olive oil with lime juice, oregano, mustard, salt, and pepper in a bowl.
4. Add tomatoes, bell pepper, olives, capers, and parsley to the oil combination, gently turning to thoroughly coat with oil mixture. Set this aside to marinate.
5. Place the cooked rice in large bowl. Combine the vegetable mixture and toss it well.
6. Garnish with diced cucumber and serve. .

Fish Veracruz

Ingredients:

- 2 pounds cold-water fish (your choice)
- 1 poblano/green pepper, diced
- 1 red pepper, diced
- 1 yellow/orange pepper, diced
- ¼ cup scallions, sliced
- ½ purple onion, diced
- 3 cloves chopped/minced garlic
- 1 cup cilantro leaves (fresh)
- 1–2 tablespoons of capers
- ½ teaspoon Celtic sea salt
- ½ teaspoon white pepper, ground
- 1 tablespoon of extra virgin olive oil
- 1 teaspoon Celtic sea salt
- 1 whole lime, freshly squeezed
- Red pepper flakes (optional)

Directions

1. Rinse the fish. Pat it dry. Using an oil mister, mist with extra virgin olive oil and sprinkle it with sea salt and pepper. Set it aside.
2. Place all of the vegetables in a bowl.
3. Add extra virgin olive oil, lime juice, Celtic sea salt, and white pepper. Mix all of the remaining ingredients together. Set aside until the fish is prepared.
4. Bake, broil, or grill the fish at two hundred degrees, until the fish is white and flaky.
5. Remove the fish and plate. Top the dish with the vegetable mixture and serve it.

Snacks

Chia Seed Energy Bar

Ingredients:

- 6 large Medjool dates
- ½ cup chia seeds
- ¼ cup shredded coconut, unsweetened
- 3 tablespoons coconut oil
- 2 teaspoons natural vanilla extract
- ¼ teaspoon cinnamon powder

Directions:

1. Remove the pits from the dates.
2. Place the dates in a food processor or blender, and pulse it several times until it forms a paste.

3. In a medium bowl, mix the date paste with the chia seeds, shredded coconut, vanilla extract, cinnamon, and coconut oil. It will form a thick dough.
4. Roll this dough into balls or press it into the bottom of a glass or silicon baking dish, and cut it into squares.
5. Place the mixture in the freezer to give it more of a chewy texture, then serve.

Green Chips

Ingredients:

- 1 bunch kale
- 1 tablespoon ghee, melted
- 1 teaspoon Celtic sea salt
- Cayenne pepper (optional, for light dusting)

Directions

1. Wash the kale leaves, and dry them in a salad spinner.
2. With a knife or kitchen shears, carefully remove the leaves from the stem.
3. Spray the kale with olive oil, and sprinkle it with seasoning salt.
4. Place this on food dehydrator trays, and dehydrate them for eight hours, or until they are crispy.

NOTE: If you don't have a food dehydrator, you can place the kale on a baking pan and bake it at three hundred degrees for ten to fifteen minutes, or until the edges turn brown (but are not burned). Remember, at this temperature, the food is highly heated, but this is still a much better alternative to potato chips.

Roasted Pumpkin Seeds

Ingredients:

- 1 ½ cups raw whole pumpkin seeds (pepitas)
- 2 teaspoons coconut oil or ghee, melted
- ½ teaspoon Celtic sea salt
- A sprinkle cayenne (optional)

Directions:

1. Melt the oil in a small skillet on medium-low heat.
2. Place the pumpkin seeds in the skillet and stir until they are coated by oil.
3. Add the sea salt (and cayenne pepper, if you like a kick). Stir to coat the seeds well and keep them in the skillet until lightly toasted. Serve.

Note: You can substitute any raw nut of your choice (except peanuts). Cinnamon may be substituted for cayenne.

Shakes and Smoothies

The following protein powders are excellent quality and cold processed:

- *Detox Plus protein powder (neuropathydoctorsa.com)*
- *SP Complete protein powder (neuropathydoctorsa.com)*
- *Raw Power and Sproutein protein powder (naturalnews.com)*
- *Miracle Whey protein powder (www.mercola.com)*

Berry Delight Shake

Ingredients

- 2 scoops of protein powder
- ¼ cup blueberries
- ¼ cup blackberries
- ¼ cup strawberries
- ½ banana
- 1 cup SO coconut milk, unsweetened
- ½ cup of apple juice, organic
- 1 teaspoon flax seed, freshly ground
- 1 cup ice *(you don't need the ice if the berries are frozen)*

Directions:

1. Place coconut milk and ice in the blender, and blend on high until the desired consistency is reached.
2. Add the rest of the ingredients, and blend it on low.
3. If the shake consistency is too thick, add some water and blend it until the desired consistency is reached.

Note: Do not confuse coconut cream with coconut milk. Coconut milk will be in the refrigerator section of the grocery store packaged in a typical half gallon milk-style carton.

Choco-Banana Shake

Ingredients:

- 2 scoops of protein powder—chocolate
- ½ banana
- 4 pieces unsweetened frozen strawberries (or your berries of choice)
- 2 ounces water
- 6 ounces coconut milk (unsweetened)
- 1 teaspoon flax seed, freshly ground
- 1 tablespoon raw honey

Directions:

1. Place six ounces of coconut milk into a blender, add the frozen fruit, and blend it to the desired consistency.
2. Add the protein powder, the ground flax, the honey, and then the water. Blend until smooth.

Foods that you should avoid:

- processed foods, fast foods, and junk foods
- sugary snacks and cereals
- soft drinks (including diet drinks)
- high fructose corn syrup
- all refined grains and wheat
- dairy products (especially those made from cow's milk, which has been shown to increase inflammation)

- vegetable oils *(sunflower, safflower, corn, grape seed)*, margarine or butter substitutes, and trans fats *(hydrogenated, or partially hydrogenated oils)*
- fried foods and all other fatty foods (fatty foods suppress the immune system and that's the last thing you need when you're fighting peripheral neuropathy.)
- processed grains and cereals
- conventionally raised meat
- processed meat
- peanuts (peanut crops have high levels of pesticide and are frequently contaminated with a carcinogenic mold called aflatoxin.);
- food additives and preservatives (MSG, Aspartame, nitrates/nitrites);
- coffee, black teas, and most caffeinated drinks (Monster, Red Bull, 5-Hour Energy, etc.);

> *Your genetics load the gun.*
> *Your lifestyle pulls the trigger.*
>
> Mehmet Oz (Dr. Oz)

- alcohol—consumption limits the ability of the liver to remove toxins from the body. Alcohol is converted to sugar.

10

MOVE IT...AND LOSE THE NEUROPATHY

"Take care of your body. It's the only place you have to live."

Jim Rohn
(1930–2009)

Exercise and Neuropathy

People suffering from neuropathy know that the pain, muscle weakness, lack of balance, and overall health complications can make everyday activities harder to manage. As previously mentioned, a person with peripheral neuropathy is often at an increased risk of experiencing falls and related injuries due to a lack of muscle control and balance. Therefore, exercise is a critical component to many therapies, since it can build muscle strength while increasing circulation and coordination. For many people, the prospect of exercising while suffering from neuropathy seems unrealistic. Immobility is a significant problem with many peripheral neuropathy patients. However, exercise is important for everyone, and it is a vital part of any recovery plan for neuropathy.

The benefits of performing appropriate exercises are extensive and far-reaching. While the general benefits of aerobic and flexibility exercises are well known, it is particularly important for people suffering with peripheral neuropathy to increase their range of motion, muscle movement, and heart rate. Physical activity can improve blood circulation, which strengthens nerve tissues by increasing the flow of oxygen.

Exercising is beneficial in maintaining control of blood sugar levels. Exercise can also minimize muscle wasting, increase muscle function by improving strength and endurance, and improve balance and mobility. According to the National Institute of Neurological Disorders and Stroke, exercise is important for individuals with peripheral neuropathy, and it can have a positive effect on your condition. The Mayo Clinic also states that exercise can help reduce neuropathy pain. Overall, exercise has been shown to actually slow down the progression and alleviate symptoms of polyneuropathy.

> **National Institutes of Health**
>
> *Exercise and diet can reduce neuropathic pain and help regenerate nerve fibers in patients with impaired glucose tolerance.*

Furthermore, exercising regularly greatly decreases anyone's risk of diabetic neuropathy, by controlling symptoms and deterioration in sufferers by elevating overall blood flow to the limbs. In fact, a recent study from the University of Utah in Salt Lake City reports that exercise and diet work hand in hand to reduce nerve pain for patients with impaired glucose tolerance and neuropathy.

The type of exercise that you choose will depend on the extent of your peripheral neuropathy and the advice of your health care professional. The dangers involved with exercising with peripheral neuropathy depend on the symptoms that you are experiencing. Some people with mild cases of the disease may be able to perform a fairly normal exercise routine, while others may need to carefully tailor their routine based on the limitations brought on by their condition.

If your muscle control and coordination are compromised, you should be concerned about possibly falling. Numbness in your feet will reduce or eliminate your ability to feel blisters, cuts, or other damage. According to the National Institute of Neurological Disorders and Stroke, if the peripheral neuropathy has affected your autonomic nerves (the ones controlling your organs and glands), you might face challenges with controlling your blood pressure, maintaining a regular heartbeat and difficulty with breathing. Additionally, autonomic nerve damage can reduce your ability to feel low blood glucose levels, which can be dangerous for diabetics.

Exercise for Mild Neuropathy

According to a 2012 study, published in the *Journal of the American Physical Therapy Association*, resistance training is a great way to improve your overall muscle strength, especially for people with diabetes and peripheral neuropathy. Participants who walked four times a week for one hour greatly diminished the progression of their peripheral neuropathy.

Researchers at the University of Louisville showed that lower-body weight training (three times a week for thirty minutes) improved muscle strength, as well as the quality of life.

These patients would perform routine tasks, such as walking to the car or getting up from a chair.

A 2006 review article published in *Alternative Medicine Review* by naturopath Kathleen Head reported that people with neuropathy who practiced yoga for thirty to forty minutes every day experienced improvements in their neuropathy symptoms. Participants experienced decreased pain levels and 40–60 percent improvements in their muscular strength.

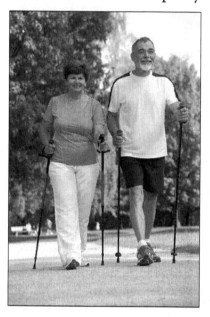

Whether your neuropathy is mild or more advanced, you should avoid high-impact exercises (*e.g.*, running on a treadmill or high-impact aerobics) because they often result in foot injuries. Some excellent choices for exercises are seated resistance exercises, which can be done with a resistance band or weights, and swimming, rowing, and pretty much any upper body exercise.

Exercise for Moderate to Severe Neuropathy

People suffering from more extensive degrees of neuropathy typically have problems with balance and muscle weakness. The National Institutes of Health (NIH) adds that the lack of sensation can result in problems determining joint position, which can lead to coordination difficulties. For these sufferers, resistance training and yoga may not be options for them.

Swimming is one of the best exercises for any age, fitness level, or degree of neuropathy symptoms. Swimming is a whole-body workout with no impact, which makes it less harmful to your joints, legs, and feet than most other forms of exercise. Furthermore, swimming increases your heart rate, which improves your circulation—a very important component for nerve regeneration. I realize that not everyone enjoys getting into the water, and not everyone is able to safely climb in and out of a pool. For these people, recumbent stationary cycling and rowing are other excellent, alterative low-impact activities that can be safely integrated into a neuropathy treatment program.

How to Begin

You should always begin any exercise session with a warm-up to avoid cramping. Slow, thirty-second sustained muscle stretching helps maintain flexibility, and it minimizes cramping during your exercises. According to Charlotte Hayes, RD, a diabetes nutrition and exercise specialist in Atlanta, (author of *The I Hate to Exercise Book for People with Diabetes*) for people who absolutely hate to exercise or simply have no extra energy, one good way to avoid muscle fatigue is to do five to ten minutes of flexibility exercises three to five times throughout the day. It is beneficial to get up once an hour to move around and stretch for even five minutes. This really does add up.

Warm-Ups and Stretching Exercises *(These can be performed seated or standing. Always keep your eyes open)*

1. Raise both of your arms straight up over your head. Stretch up and through your fingertips. Next, lean as far

as you can to the right, with arms still overhead, and hold it for twenty seconds. Slowly return to the center. Next, lean as far as you can to the left and hold for twenty seconds. Return to the center and relax.

2. Raise your arms overhead once again and lean forward from the waist as far as you can without getting uncomfortable or losing your balance. Hold for twenty seconds and return to the starting position. Lower your arms and relax.

3. Lift both of your arms straight out to the sides like someone is stretching you in a tug of war. Keep your feet facing forward. Rotate only your upper body at the waist to the right and hold for twenty seconds. Return to the center. Next, rotate to the left and hold for twenty seconds, and then return to center.

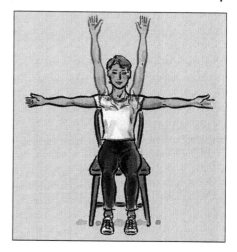

Hand and Finger Exercises:

1. Touch the tip of your thumb to the tip of your index finger, making a round circle like an OK sign. Stretch the

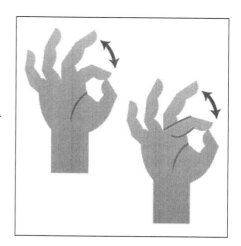

hand open. Repeat this with your middle, ring, and little finger in succession.
2. Touch the pad of your thumb with the pad of your index finger. Move your index finger down to the base of your thumb. Repeat twice with your index, middle, ring, and little fingers in succession.
3. Place the palms of your hands on your lap. Lift your index finger three times, and tap your lap. Repeat this twice with each finger in succession.
4. Clasp your hands loosely together. Circle your thumbs around each other ten times in a clockwise direction, and then reverse and circle your fingers ten times in a counterclockwise direction.

Seated Exercises for Neuropathy Involving the Feet, Ankles, and Legs:

1. Keeping your heels on the floor, gently raise your toes up as high as possible. Then, lower your toes back to the floor and gently tap several times with the toes.

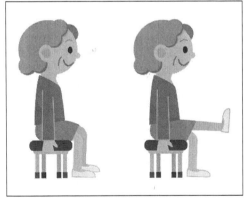

2. Keeping your heels together on the floor, lift your toes off the floor as high as possible. Turn your toes out so that your foot forms a V. Then place your feet back on the floor. Next, lift your

toes again, bring them together, and put them back on the floor. Repeat this five times.
3. With your knees together, lift your right foot off the floor while straightening your knee at the same time. Point your toe toward the floor and then flex your ankle with your toe pointed toward the ceiling. Repeat this five times. Last, circle your ankle clockwise and then counterclockwise five times each. Repeat this on the other side.
4. Raise both of your heels off the floor at the same time, as if you are standing on your tiptoes. Hold for twenty seconds and then slowly lower down. Repeat this five times.

Balance Exercises:

Balance and coordination commonly become impaired in neuropathy sufferers, causing instability. This leads to high incidences of falls. Problems with walking and balancing arise when a person experiences a decrease in sensory input. The diminished sensation can interfere with their ability to determine where their legs and feet are in space, causing a person to stumble or fall. People with peripheral neuropathy might experience awkward foot positioning due to a lack of muscle control, sudden shifts in positioning—altering their center of gravity—and a lack of feeling in the feet, resulting in changes in walking patterns and imbalance.

Those who exercise will improve their balance, flexibility, and coordination, and they will have a reduced risk of falling.

When you work on balance exercises, it is very important that you are cautious so you do not fall. It may be necessary for a person to assist or supervise to prevent you from falling. You may use a walker, if one is available, to steady yourself. If your balance is good enough, you can stand behind a sturdy chair.

1. March gently in place, lifting only your heels off the floor. When this becomes easy, lift your heels and toes off of the floor, very slightly, as you march in place. As your balance improves, lift your feet higher off the floor. *Variation: if you are too unsteady, you can perform this exercise while seated.*
2. Stand slowly up on your tiptoes, and then go back on your heels. Do not lock your knees. Repeat this five times.
3. [*More advanced*] Step to the side with your right foot, and then bring your left foot next to your right foot. Next, step to the side with the left foot, and then bring your right foot next to it. Repeat this several times. As your balance improves, take larger steps to the side.
4. Stand up tall. Keeping your torso straight up and down and your feet flat on the floor, bend your knees and your hips slightly, sinking down into a squatting position. Then, straighten your hips and knees and stand back up- straight. Repeat this several times. If you

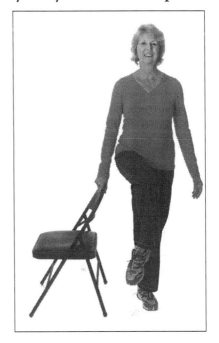

experience knee pain, stand up to point at which you don't have the pain. Do not bend or squat past this level. As your balance and strength improve, bend your knees a little bit more *(if your knee pain persists, stop the exercise)*.

In addition to its physical benefits, exercise can also improve your mental health and overall mood. Regular exercise reduces the amount of stress hormones that your body releases, and it increases the amount of endorphins. Endorphins are chemicals in the brain that are referred to as happy hormones because they elevate your mood and act as a powerful pain-reliever. Give your body time to get adjusted to your exercise routine. After just a few weeks of incorporating these new movements, you'll wind up feeling relaxed and refreshed. Most people even notice that their sleep improves.

> **Five signs of excessive exercise**
>
> 1. Feeling weaker, rather than stronger, after thirty minutes of exercise;
> 2. Excessive muscle soreness twenty-four to forty-eight hours after exercise;
> 3. Severe muscle cramping;
> 4. Heaviness in the extremities
> 5. Prolonged shortness of breath.

11

TAKE BACK CONTROL

"It is not that some people do not know what to do with truth when it is offered to them, but the tragic fate is a condition of mind-blindness, in which the truth is not recognized, though it stares you in the face."

Sir William Oster, Physician
(1849–1919)

If you have made it this far into the book, I congratulate you for taking the time and effort to become more informed about your health. Your head may be spinning with what is new and potentially life-altering information. You might be laden at this very moment with mixed emotions—emotions roiling deep down in your gut that may be simultaneously conjuring up fear and excitement. How can you be experi-

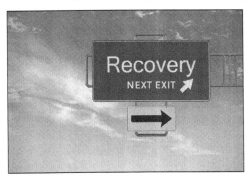

encing these two emotions on opposite ends of the spectrum? It is because you are about to make a paradigm shift.

A paradigm is a model or a concept of something. It can also be a typical (sometimes stereotypical) example of something. They are a necessary part of our thought process, but they can also create obstacles.

Paradigms are the lens through which we view our world and ourselves. They are a set of rules and regulations that establishes and defines boundaries for you. Paradigms tell you how to behave inside these boundaries. For example, decades ago, a common paradigm was for a mother to give up work to raise a family while the father went out to earn a living. The male figure in a marriage was considered to be the breadwinner, while the female's role was that of the homemaker.

Paradigms are the sum of our basic concepts, values, traditions, principles, prejudices, rituals, and superstitions that formulate a way of viewing reality for the community that shares them. If our paradigms are incorrect, then we will have incorrect thoughts, actions, and results. A powerful example of the limiting effect of a wrong paradigm was when people believed that the world was flat and that if they travelled too far they would fall off the edge. This incorrect paradigm limited exploration for a very long time.

A paradigm shift is when the usual and accepted way of doing or thinking about something is changed. Think of a paradigm shift as a change from one way of thinking to another. It is a transformation and a metamorphosis. One example of a paradigm shift was the widely accepted thought that the human body was not capable of running a four-minute mile. How did this become a paradigm? For nine consecutive years, no one was able to break the one-mile record of 4 minutes, 1.4

seconds until May 6, 1954. Roger Bannister said, "It didn't seem logical to me, as a physiologist/doctor, that if you could run a mile in four minutes, one and a bit seconds, you couldn't break four minutes." He changed the paradigm forever by running one mile in 3 minutes, 59.4 seconds. He changed the psychological and physical barrier that had been created, thus causing a paradigm shift. Amazingly enough, once this shift had been created sixteen other runners ran a four-minute mile within the next three years.

Why am I spending time talking about paradigms and shifts? A number of myths have been debunked—myths that you have accepted as your reality, your paradigm. Based on all that you have learned from reading this book, many of you will need to prepare yourself to make a paradigm shift in your health. This sounds simple, but I do want to prepare you. When a paradigm becomes subconscious, it begins to define the reality of personal experience, thus making it more difficult to replace. Therefore, when we must change a paradigm it can cause anxiety and confusion. This is a common reaction so don't be alarmed.

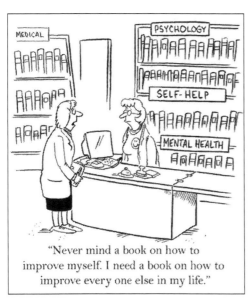

"Never mind a book on how to improve myself. I need a book on how to improve every one else in my life."

You should now realize that you are not helpless, and you can take the necessary steps to start the healing process. To come this far and not make the shift would be to remain paralyzed and imprisoned in a state of chronic illness. Right now you are probably wondering, "Where do I begin?" Or you may still be stuck in your old paradigm. The paradigm that may have been cemented into you through chronic repetition is, "You must learn to live with your neuropathy." This paradigm is *wrong*! Just like the fact that the world is not flat. It is time for you to make the paradigm shift for yourself. Remember, information without action is useless.

You can begin to make changes today. Often, the biggest obstacle to your recovery is you. We may become blind to many of our observations when they do not fit our expectations. For instance, I have watched multiple patients create their own self-fulfilling prophesy of failure. I had a patient who noticed that her neuropathy symptoms were diminishing, substantially. She began to experience an increase in energy and the ability to become more active. Unfortunately, this patient had a well-intentioned person telling her, "Be careful, this is only temporary. *My* doctor says that your nerves can't heal and you are going to need medication." I can't begin to tell you how powerful those negative words were for my patient. Even though she had seen and experienced for herself the remarkable improvement, she fell back into her old paradigm. And guess what? Her condition, once again, began to deteriorate.

The mind is a powerful thing. The change, **your change**, must begin in your mind. You need to change the way you think, which might mean changing your belief system—your paradigm. **You need to conceive it and believe it. Then you can achieve it.** This is a paradigm shift.

This book has provided you with ample information and research to empower you to say, "Yes, it's possible to defeat neuropathy, in spite of what my doctor tells me. There are other options than medications, and yes, my nerves will regenerate with the proper tools and action!" You could spend a lifetime researching the information provided in this book, but at some point, you have to take action. The sooner you take action, the better.

"It becomes obvious that if we want to make relatively minor changes in our lives, we can perhaps appropriately focus on our attitudes and behaviors. But if we want to make significant, quantum change, we need to work on our basic paradigms." ~ Stephen Covey, author of *The Seven Habits of Highly Effective People*

You can apply this principle to your health. It is the health paradigm shift that you or your loved one may very well need. Once you discover new and valid information about health and wellness, you will want to change the way you handle health challenges for you and your loved ones.

Paradigm Blindness

Sometimes we can be blind to new paradigms that may lead to devastating results.

Western Union once suffered from such blindness. An internal memo from 1876 stated, "The telephone has too many shortcomings to be seriously considered as a means of communication. The device is inherently of no value to us." This paradigm paralysis cost Western Union dearly, while paving the way for Ma Bell. I hear that Ma Bell was extremely grateful to Western Union for its ignorance.

It's easy to find excuses for why you can't take control of your health. For instance, some people say, "I can't take any supplements because I have to show my doctor everything that I take." Have you ever stopped to wonder how many hours of education your doctor had on nutrition and supplementation? Try less than ten hours, on average. You typically get better advice on nutrition from a GNC clerk than from the average doctor.

There will always be obstacles to anything that you want to accomplish in life, whether it involves your health, career, marriage, or anything else. You must learn to create your own paradigm shift.

Creating Your Own Paradigm Shifts

Now that we understand what a paradigm is and realize that we need to create a paradigm shift that aligns with our health goals, here's what you need to do:

1. <u>Set health goals</u>: Make a decision to change any paradigm that doesn't align with your ideals.
2. <u>Get out of your own way:</u> Break free from negativity. Don't let worry or fear stand in the way of your recovery. Develop a positive attitude even if you have to fake it at first. You know the old saying: "Fake it until you can make it!" Do not allow yourself to be influenced by others' negativity.
3. <u>Always use the word</u> *when:* In your conversation, instead of saying, "*If* I recover," say, "*When* I recover from this neuropathy, I will…" *(You get to fill in the blank—make it fun!)*

4. <u>Visualize your recovery</u>: Picture yourself whole again and completely healed. Mentally preview the steps necessary to reach your health goal, and then envision your day without any pain or limitations. (Many Olympic gold-medal athletes will spend as much time working on the visualization of the steps leading them to that gold-medal platform as they spend actually training. They will picture each step and movement followed by victory. You need to do this as well.)
5. <u>Make your self-talk positive</u>: Self-talk is what you say or think to yourself, either silently or aloud. Every thought will either move you toward your goal or push you away from your goal. Positive self-talk is based on thoughts that you intentionally choose to think because they will move you toward accomplishing your health goal. Tell yourself, "Others have healed from neuropathy and so can I!" As King Solomon said, "For as he thinks within himself, so he is." (Proverbs 23:7 NIV)
6. <u>Use positive affirmations</u>: Create a positive affirmation, a short powerful statement, that is opposite your current paradigm—or at least consistent with your desired results—to create a paradigm shift. It should be stated positively in the present tense. An example of a good positive affirmation is: "I have the power to take control of my health. My nerves are healing, and I am healthy again. I am not allowing any person to stand in the way of my recovery. I am doing all that is necessary to feel good and reclaim my health and my life."

Positive Affirmations + Positive Self-Talk + Repetition + Time = Paradigm Shift

Stephen Covey states in his book *The Seven Habits of Highly Effective People*, "Each of us tends to think we see things as they are, that we are objective. But this is not the case. We see the world, not as it is, but as we are—or as we are conditioned to see it."

> *It always seems impossible until it is done.*
> Nelson Mandela

12

FORMULATING A GAME PLAN

"We are what we repeatedly do. Excellence, therefore, is not an act but a habit."

Aristotle
(384–322 BC)

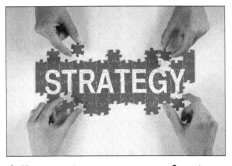

Let's review the things that you can do to begin your journey to recovery. In some cases, these are not things that you need to do but rather things that you need to stop doing that are sabotaging your health. However, the following is a summary of actions you can begin to take today:

1. Eat a whole-food diet.

A whole-food diet refers to eating fresh food that is full of life and has not been processed. This would exclude anything that comes from a box, bag, or can. Your diet should include plenty of fruits, vegetables, seeds, nuts, organic free-range poultry, wild fish, and legumes. Ideally you should purchase meat, fruits, and vegetables that are organic. However, if this is not feasible, you should at least avoid the produce with the highest levels of pesticide residue, which is known as the dirty dozen, or you should buy organic if you decide to consume the foods on this list. Visit our website, www.neuropathydoctorsa.com, to print a wallet-sized list of the dirty dozen to take with you to the grocery store.

2. Take neurotrophic supplements.

Neurotropic supplements are concentrated, whole-food-derived nutrients that are beneficial for the nervous system. In other words, they are specific nutrients that support repair and regeneration of the damaged nerves. The list of nutrients that play a critical role in the healing process is rather extensive and it can be overwhelming. This list includes: alpha lipoic acid, vitamins C and E, N-Acetylcysteine (NAC), gamma-linolenic acid (GLA), Omega-3s, and Vitamins B1, B3, B5, B6, and B12.

My patients often bring in neuropathy formulations that they have purchased on the Internet. The directions are to take two capsules, twice per day. It's virtually impossible to condense a capsule with all of the required nutrients in the proper therapeutic dosage down to two capsules that are taken twice daily. This is evident by the abysmal results reported from my patients. However, the alternative of having a cabinet filled with seven or eight different supplement bottles that you need to take daily can be daunting.

For our patients, Dr. Coppola and I have created a formulation that combines a synergistic blend of nutrients in the appropriate therapeutic doses to achieve and support nerve repair and regeneration. We have named it *NEURO-GEN*. Visit www.neuropathydoctorsa.com to learn more.

3. Start exercising.

If you don't use it, you lose it. This certainly holds true with neuropathy. When you remain sedentary, you will suffer from accelerated loss of balance, muscle strength, and cardiovascular fitness. Ideally, you should be walking for thirty minutes, four to five times per week. It is important to do a whole-body-stretching program with the same frequency. Depending on your level of stability and severity of neuropathy, a rebounder (a mini-trampoline) is an excellent form of exercise (this is typically best with mild-to-moderate neuropathy but not with severe cases). If your condition does not permit you to walk, then you can exercise while seated in a chair, swimming in a pool, or even lying on a bed. For more information, please see the previous chapter.

4. Reduce medications with medical supervision.

As you have seen in previous chapters, medications have serious side effects. Many of the medications that you are taking might be contributing to your neuropathy. I have seen far too many patients walk into my clinic slurring their speech—or appearing *zombied-out*—because they are overmedicated. Reducing your medications is, by far, one of the single best things you can do for your overall health. Talk to your doctors about a strategy to correct the medical problem that is causing your symptoms in the first place. Once this is done, your doctor can begin to reduce or eliminate many of your medications. Are you on several medications for one problem? For example, are you taking three different types of blood pressure medications? If so, talk to your doctor to find out if all three are necessary. Seek natural health care providers to find alternatives to medications.

5. Drink purified water daily.

Although you would think this would be a no-brainer, the reality is that 75 percent of the population is chronically dehydrated. Do not drink tap water! My first choice is good quality spring water or otherwise filtered water. The general rule of thumb is to drink half of your body weight in ounces. For example, if you weight 150 pounds, drink 75 ounces of water per day. And no, coffee doesn't count. Remember, coffee is a diuretic and it will cause you to lose your precious minerals. For a good water filtration system, visit: www.aquasana.com or www.stpaulmercantile.com (type in stainless steel water filter).

6. Start juicing.

Buy a juicer and use it. We live in a day and age when our soil is overcultivated. We eat too much processed food, and we destroy any remaining nutrients by storing our food for too long or by overcooking it. Suffice it to say, we are all nutrient-deficient to some degree. One of the best ways to restore nutritional deficiencies is to juice on a regular basis (weekly). Fresh juice is supercharged with antioxidants, enzymes, vitamins, and minerals. It will deliver necessary nutrients to your cells and nerves for healing, and your energy levels will increase. For people with prediabetes or diabetes, I recommend using a Vitamix turbo blender as opposed to a juicer. The Vitamix retains all of the fiber from your fruits and vegetables, lowering the glycemic index and preventing a fast sugar dump into the bloodstream. (visit www.harvestessentials.com or www.costco.com).

7. Detox.

Detoxing is like spring-cleaning for the body. Impurities, such as accumulated chemicals and toxins, are removed from the blood in the liver, where toxins are processed for elimination. A detox program should be done minimally once per year–every year. A typical detox program will include dietary alterations, which does not necessarily mean fasting, along with specific nutritional supplements designed to aid and support the toxin removal from the body. I recommend a four-week detox program, but if you are new to detoxing, you can start with two to three 10 day detoxes throughout the year. You can consult a natural health care provider or seek out a detox book that is right for you.

8. Avoid MSG and artificial sweeteners.

MSG and artificial sweeteners (the blue, pink, and yellow packets) are neurotoxins—not exactly what you want to be eating when you're trying to recover from neuropathy. Hence, avoid zero-calorie soda drinks—or any soda drink, for that matter. Read the labels carefully. Never, ever, ever, eat anything without scrutinizing the label first—not unless you like playing Russian roulette with your health.

9. Get at least thirty minutes of sun exposure daily.

With all of the hoopla about skin cancer, people are avoiding sun exposure entirely. Don't get me wrong, we must use common sense and avoid overexposure; however, thirty minutes of sun exposure daily is extremely beneficial to your health. We have an epidemic of vitamin D deficiency. So, take a daily walk in the sun for thirty minutes. By the way, ditch the sunscreen for those thirty minutes. Sunscreen inhibits the production of vitamin D.

10. Stop smoking!

With all of the data that conclusively proves that smoking causes cancer, it amazes me that people continue to smoke. Smoking is especially harmful to someone trying to recover from neuropathy. Smoking reduces oxygenation to the cells and it impairs circulation.

11. Seek a neuropathy doctor who specializes in nonsurgical, drug-free treatments.

Even Michael Jordan had a coach. If you have committed to all of the steps in this book, and you are not getting the results that you had hoped for, then it's time to seek professional assistance. To fast-track your recovery, I recommend taking all of the steps in this book while working with a health professional. To guide you in selecting a health professional, see the recommended guidelines below.

12. Be 1000 percent committed to your recovery!

Commitment is the resolution to do whatever it takes to achieve your goal. Without commitment, you will not take the necessary actions. Even if you take some actions, without absolute commitment you will not persevere long enough to achieve the desired results. It is much easier to do nothing and wallow in pain and sorrow, but in the end a much greater price will be paid – the loss of your health. The steps outlined in this book will take invested time, energy, and resources—but then again, all great accomplishments do.

> *"It is not enough that we do our best; sometimes we must do what is required."*
>
> Winston Churchill
> (1874-1965)

SELECTING A HEALTH PROFESSIONAL FOR NEUROPATHY CARE

Six questions to consider before beginning a treatment program for neuropathy:

1. Has a thorough, in-depth evaluation and examination been performed to diagnose my nerve dysfunction?
2. Does the treatment address the cause(s) of my neuropathy and not just the pain?
3. Does the treatment reduce inflammation not only at the nerve but throughout the body?
4. Does the treatment increase the cellular ATP production that is necessary for nerve repair and healing?
5. Does the treatment use neurotrophic nutrients to promote nerve repair and regeneration?
6. Does the treatment reestablish the communication between the damaged peripheral nerves and the brain?

We're not going to achieve real health if we're just tackling symptoms instead of addressing the underlying causes. There must be a health paradigm shift that changes the way we see things, changes the way we behave, and changes our attitudes toward health and life in general.

"If you do what you've always done, you'll get what you've always gotten. For changes to be of any true value, they've got to be lasting and consistent." ~ Tony Robbins

Polyneuropathy does not have to be something that you are forced to live with. Neuropathy is indeed reversible! I have a saying: "There is no unrealistic goal—only unrealistic time frames." The degree of involvement and effort required to resolve your neuropathy is dependent on the number of contributing variables or causes and the amount of time you have been inflicted with neuropathy. However, it is imperative to have all of the necessary ingredients in the treatment recipe to heal the nerves and reverse this condition.

It's important to remember that neuropathy can affect people of all ages. Some of my younger neuropathy patients have been in their thirties, but by far the most common cases affect patients in their sixties and higher. After reading this book, you should be able to make sense of your condition and its effects. By this stage of life, many of you have been exposed to neuropathy-causing factors for many years. This is sad and unfortunate, as this condition will rob you of what should be your golden years.

The most fulfilling part of my career is being able to help people recover from neuropathy and return to their normal lives. Some of my patients had previously given up the activities that they loved the most, such as gardening, golfing, playing with their grandchildren, horseback riding, or just taking a stroll through the mall. After undergoing our comprehensive treatment program for neuropathy, they were able to return to all of their favorite activities.

Remember...*You Don't Have To Live With Neuropathy!*

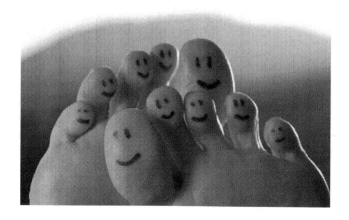

> *The healing journey that you are about to embark on is not a burden or a chore, but a blessing. It will be your greatest adventure inward to discover and create a new healthy life!*
>
> Dr. Richard Schulze

Neuropathydoctorsa.com

GLOSSARY

Advanced glycation end products (AGEs): the end products of glycation reactions, in which a sugar molecule bonds to either a protein or lipid (fat) molecule without an enzyme to control the reaction. Without the enzyme to control the reaction, glycation occurs haphazardly impairing normal functioning of molecules. This can lead to carcinogenic and toxic damage to a number of cells.

Anoxia: a condition characterized by an absence of oxygen supply to an organ or a tissue.

Arrhythmia: any abnormality in the rhythm of the heartbeat.

Atrophy: a wasting or decrease in size of a body organ, tissue, or part owing to disease, degeneration of cells, injury, or lack of use.

Autonomic nervous system (ANS): part of the peripheral nervous system that controls involuntary organ functions, such as breathing, heart rate, digestion, urination, etc.

Axon: the long slender projection of a nerve cell (also known as a nerve fiber) that conducts electrical impulses away from the nerve.

Blood-brain barrier (BBB): a filtering mechanism composed of high-density capillary cells that restricts the passage of some harmful substances, such as bacteria and chemicals, while allowing nutrient-like substances to enter freely.

Catalyst: a substance that increases the rate of a chemical reaction without itself undergoing any permanent chemical change.

Central nervous system (CNS): the brain and spinal cord.

Cerebrospinal fluid (CSF): a clear, watery fluid that is continuously produced and flows within the brain, around the outer surface of the brain, and through the spinal cord. Its main function is to protect the brain and spinal cord by acting as a shock absorber to cushion or absorb the impact of a fall or blow to the head. It also removes waste and circulates nutrients within the CNS.

Constrict: to make smaller or narrower, especially by compressing or squeezing.

Cytosol: the solution of proteins and metabolites inside a biological cell.

Demyelination: a partial or complete breakdown in the myelin sheath.

Dendrite: a branched projection of a nerve that receives signals from the brain and spinal cord and sends the messages down the axon (nerve fiber).

Diabetes: a chronic illness in which a person has high blood sugar, either because the body does not produce enough insulin, or because cells do not respond to the insulin that is produced.

Dilate: to become wider or larger; to expand.

Electrolyte: a solution that conducts electricity.

Electromyography: a diagnostic technique that is used for evaluating and recording the electrical activity produced by skeletal muscles.

Endorphins: a group of hormones found mainly in the brain that bind to opiate receptors to reduce the sensation of pain and elevate your mood; the body's natural painkillers.

Environmental toxin: any potentially harmful substance that contaminates the air, water, or land.

Epidermis: the outer nonvascular layer of skin, which is made up of five layers and lies on top of the dermis.

Excitotoxin: glutamate and other similar substances that create a pathological process by which nerve cells are damaged and killed.

Fasciculation: muscular twitching involving the simultaneous contraction of contiguous groups of muscle fibers.

Glucose: a simple sugar that cells within the human body use as a primary source of energy.

Hyponatremia: abnormally low level of sodium in the blood; associated with dehydration.

Insulin: a hormone secreted by the pancreas that is necessary for the metabolism of carbohydrates and the regulation of glucose levels in the blood.

Innervate: to arouse or stimulate a nerve or an organ to activity.

Kombucha: a raw fermented tea made from symbiotic (probiotic) cultures of bacteria and yeast and containing natural effervescence.

Lipid: any of a group of organic compounds that are greasy to the touch, insoluble in water, and soluble in alcohol and ether: lipids comprise the fats and other esters with analogous properties and constitute, with proteins and carbohydrates, the chief structural components of living cells.

Macrobiotic diet: first mentioned in the writings of Hippocrates, the term *macrobiotic* translates as "great life." The foods incorporated into this diet are organic whole foods, including fruits, fresh vegetables, sea vegetables, legumes, whole grains, and raw nuts. Fish and meat are consumed very minimally. All processed foods are avoided. The diet focuses on low fat.

Metabolite: a substance that is essential to a particular metabolic process; for example, glucose is a metabolite of sugars and starches, and amino acids are metabolites of proteins.

Mononeuropathy: damage affecting a single nerve that resides outside of the brain and spinal cord.

Motor nerves: nerves that send impulses from the brain and spinal cord to all muscles in the body.

Myelin sheath: a protective coating, made up of proteins and fat, around the axon (nerve fiber) that serves as a protection to the nerve, preventing the interference of signals or crosstalk between nerves. Also, this speeds up the rate of nerve transmission.

Nervous system: a network of nerve cells that transmits signals to and from the brain, spinal cord, and peripheral nerves.

Nerve conduction study (NCS): **a** test that is commonly used to evaluate the function and ability of electrical conduction of the motor and sensory nerves of the human body.

Neuron: an electrically excitable nerve cell that processes and transmits information along the nervous system.

Neurodegeneration: the progressive loss of function and structure, or death, of nerve cells or neurons.

Neurodegenerative disease: an umbrella term describing a range of conditions caused by the loss of function, structure, or death of a nerve cell or neuron. Examples include Alzheimer's, Parkinson's, and Huntington's diseases.

Neurotoxin: a chemical or substance that inhibits the functions of nerves or causes damage to nerves.

Neurotransmitter: A chemical substance that is released at the end of a nerve fiber by the arrival of a nerve impulse and by diffusing across the synapse or junction causes the transfer of the impulse to another nerve fiber, a muscle fiber, or some other structure.

Paresthesia: a sensation of prickling, tingling, or creeping on the skin that has no known cause.

Peripheral nervous system (PNS): nerves that extend outside of the brain and spinal cord, serving organs and limbs.

Peripheral neuritis: inflammation of several peripheral nerves simultaneously.

Peripheral neuropathy: damage or disease of the nerves that reside outside of the brain and spinal cord. This is most prevalent in the limbs.

Polyneuropathy: damage affecting multiple nerves that reside outside of brain and spinal cord.

Polyneuritis: inflammation of several peripheral nerves simultaneously, *also known as peripheral neuritis.*

Proprioceptor: special nerve endings in the muscles, tendons, and organs that respond to stimuli regarding the position and movement of the body.

Quantitative sensory testing (QST): a method used to assess damage in both small and large nerve endings, which detect changes in temperature and vibration.

Sensory nerves: nerves that receive sensory stimuli (sharp, rough, smooth, burning, etc.) and send these messages from the muscles or skin back to the spinal cord and brain.

Synapse: a structure that permits a nerve cell to pass an electrical or chemical signal to another cell within the body.

Synaptic junction: a gap in nerve cells that permits the neuron to pass an electrical or chemical signal across a gap to another nerve cell.

Toxin: a substance or chemical created by artificial (industrial) processes that can be absorbed into the body and is capable of causing disease.

Neuropathydoctorsa.com

FOOTNOTES and PERIPHERAL NEUROPATHY REFERENCES

Footnotes

1-5. *Consumer Reports Best Buy Drugs: Shoppers Guide to Prescription Drugs*, No. 6: Off-Label Drug Use.
6. *The Merck Manual of Diagnosis and Therapy*, 19th edition.
7. Weimer L.H., "Medication-Induced Peripheral Neuropathy," *Curr. Neurol. Neurosci. Rep.* Jan 2003(1):86-92..

Peripheral Neuropathy References

Abernathy, C. O., et al. "Arsenic: Health Effects, Mechanisms of Actions, and Research Issues." *Environ. Health Perspect.* 107 (1999): 593-597.
Abuaisha, B. B., Costanzi, J. B., & Boulton, A. J. (1998). "Acupuncture for the Treatment of Chronic Painful Peripheral Diabetic Neuropathy: A Long-Term Study." *Diabetes Research and Clinical Practice* 39(2) (1998): 115–121.
Alberti, K. G., et al. "Harmonizing the Metabolic Syndrome: A Joint Interim Statement of the International Diabetes Federation Task Force on Epidemiology and Prevention: National Heart, Lung, and Blood Institute; American Heart Association; World Heart Federation; International Atherosclerosis Society; and International Association for the Study of Obesity. *Circulation* 120 (2009): 1640-1645.
Alliance for Human Research Protection. "Pfizer Lawsuits: Zoloft/Neurontin Concealed Evidence: Suicide Risk/ Lack of Efficacy" , http://www.ahrp.org, July 26, 2004.
Berenson, A. "Cholesterol Drug has No Benefit in Trial. *New York Times.* Jan 14, 2008.
Culver, A. L., et al. "Statin Use and Risk of Diabetes Mellitus in Postmenopausal Women in the Women's Health Initia-

tive." *Arch. Intern. Med.* 172(2) (2012): 144–152. doi:10.1001/archinternmed.2011.625.

Appel, L.J., Moore, T.J., Obarzaneck, E., et al. "A Clinical Trial of the Effects of Dietary Patterns on Blood Pressure. DASH Collaborative Research Group." *New England Journal of Medicine* 336 (1997): 1117–1124.

Argyriou, A. A., Chroni, E., Koutras, A., Ellul, J., Papapetropoulos, S., Katsoulas, G., et al. "Vitamin E for Prophylaxis Against Chemotherapy-Induced Neuropathy." *Neurology* 64(1) (2005): 26–31.

Armstrong, T., Almadrones, L., & Gilbert, M. Chemotherapy-induced peripheral neuropathy. *Oncology Nursing Forum* 32(2) (2005): 305–311.

Araki, S., Honma, T. "Relationships Between Lead Absorption and Peripheral Nerve Conduction Verocities In Lead Workers." Scand. J. Work Environ. & Health 4 (1976): 225–31.

Araki, S., Yokoyama, K., Murata, K. "Assessment of the Effects of Occupational and Environmental Factors on All Faster and Slower Large Myelinated Nerve Fibers. A Study of the Distribution of Nerve Conduction Velocities." *Environ. Res.* 62 (1993b): 325–32.

Arnall, D. A., Nelson, A. G., Lopez, L., Sanz, M., Iversen, L., Sanz, I., et al.. "The Restorative Effects of Pulsed Infrared Light Therapy on Significant Loss of Peripheral Protective Sensation in Patients With Long-Term Type 1 and Type 2 Diabetes Mellitus." *Acta Diabetologica* 43(1) (2006): 26–33.

Ashton-Miller, J., Yeh, M., Richardson, J. K., & Galloway, T. (1996). "A Cane Reduces Loss of Balance in Patients With Peripheral Neuropathy: Results From a Challenging Unipedal Balance Test." *Archives of Physical Medicine and Rehabilitation* 77(5), (1996): 446–452.

Attal, N., et al. "EFNS Guidelines on Pharmacological Treatment of Neuropathic Pain." *Eur. J. Neurology* 13 (2006):1153–1169.

Avorn, J. *Powerful Medicines: The Benefits, Risks, and Costs of Prescription Drugs.* Random House, 2004.

Balducci, S., Iacobellis, G., Parisi, L., Di Biase, N., Calandriello, E., Leonetti, F., et al. Exercise Training Can Modify the Natural History of Diabetic Peripheral Neuropathy. *Journal of Diabetes and Its Complications,* 20(4) (2006): 216–223.

Bianchi, G., Vitali, A., Ravaglia, S., Capri, G., Cundari, S., Zanna, C., et al. Symptomatic and Neurophysiological Responses of Paclitaxel or Cisplatin-Induced Neuropathy to Oral Acetyl-L-Carnitine." *European Journal of Cancer* 41(12) (2005): 1746–1750.

Bo, S., Durazzo, M., Gambino, R., Berutti, C. and Milanesio, N., et al. "Associations of Dietary and Serum Copper With Inflammation, Oxidative Stress and Metabolic Variables in Adults." *J. Nutr.* 138 (2008): 305–10. PMID: 18203896

Bove, L., Picardo, M., Maresca, V., Jaredolo, B., & Pace, A. "A Pilot Study on the Relation Between Cisplatin Neuropathy and Vitamin E." *Journal of Experimental and Clinical Cancer Research* 20(2), (2001): 277–280.

Brucker-Davis, F. "Effects of Environmental Synthetic Chemicals on Thyroid Function." *Thyroid* 8 (1998): 827–56.

Cascinu, S., Catalano, V., Cordella, L., Labiance, R., Giordani, P., Baldelli, A.M., et al. "Neuroprotective Effect of Reduced Glutathione on Oxaliplatin-Based Chemotherapy in Advanced Colorectal Cancer: A Randomized, Double-

Blind, Placebo-Controlled Trial." *Journal of Clinical Oncology* 20(16) (2002): 3478–3483.

Cascinu, S., Cordella, L., Del Ferro, E., Fronzoni, M., & Catalana, G. (1995). Neuroprotective Effect of Reduced Glutathione on Cisplatin-Based Chemotherapy in Advanced Gastric Cancer: A Randomized, Double-Blind, Placebo-Controlled Trial." *Journal of Clinical Oncology* 13(1) (1995): 26–32.

Caspersen, C. J., Powell, K. E., & Christenson, G. M. (1985). "Physical Activity, Exercise and Physical Fitness: Definitions and Distinctions for Health Related Research. *Public Health Reports* 100 (1985): 126–131. PubMed Abstract.

Cata, J. P., Cordella, J. V., Burton, A. W., Hassenbusch, S. J., Weng, H. R., & Dougherty, P. M. "Spinal Cord Stimulation Relieves Chemotherapy-Induced Pain: A Clinical Case Report." *Journal of Pain and Symptom Management* 27(1) (2004): 72–78.

Chai, J., Herrmann, D. N., Stanton, M., Barbano, R. L., Logigian, E. "Painful Small-Fiber Neuropathy in Sjogren Syndrome." *Neurology* 65 (2005): 925–927

Chun LJ, Tong MJ, Busuttil RW, Hiatt JR,."Acetaminophen hepatotoxicity and acute liver failure." J Clin Gastroenterol. 2009 Apr;43(4):342-9.

David Preiss et al. (2011). Risk of Incident Diabetes With Intensive-Dose Compared With Moderate-DoseStatin Therapy: A Meta-analysis JAMA. 2011;305(24):2556-2564. doi: 10.1001/jama.2011.860

Davis, I. D., Kiers, L., MacGregor, L., Quinn, M., Arezo, J., Green, M., et al. "A Randomized, Double-Blind, Placebo-Controlled Phase II Trial of Recombinant Human Leukemia Inhibitory Factor (rhuLIF, emfilermin, AMg424) to

Prevent Chemotherapy-Induced Peripheral Neuropathy." *Clinical Cancer Research* 11(5), (2005): 1890–1898.

Eckel, F., Schmelz, R., Adelsberger, H., Erdmann, J., Quasthoff, F., & Lersch, C. [Prevention of Oxaliplatin-Induced Neuropathy by Carbamazepine: A Pilot Study]. *Deutsche Medizinische Wochenschrift* 127(3) (2002): 78–82.

El-Nabarawy, S. K., El-Gelel Mohamed, M. A., Ahmed, M. M., El-Arabi, G. H., "Alpha-Lipoic Acid Therapy Modulates Serum Levels of Some Trace Elements and Antioxidants in Type 2 Diabetic Patients." *Am.J. Pharm. & Toxicol.* 5(3) (2010): 152–158.

Fengsheng, H. (2000) "Neurotoxic Effects of Insecticides, Current and Future Research: A Review." *NeuroToxicol* 21 (2000): 829–36.

Flatters, S., Xiao, W. & Bennett, G.J. (2006). "Acetyl-L-Carnitine Prevents and Reduces Paclitaxel-Induced Painful Peripheral Neuropathy." *Neuroscience Letters* 397 (2006): 219–223. PubMed Abstract.

Forst, T., Nguyen, M., Forst, S., Disselhoff, B., Pohlmann, T., & Pfutzner, A. (2004). "Impact of Low Frequency Transcutaneous Electrical Nerve Stimulation on Symptomatic Diabetic Neuropathy Using the New Salutaris Device. *Diabetes, Nutrition and Metabolism* 17(3) (2004): 163–168.

Franz, J. Ingelfinger, MD: Dorlands Medical Dictionary, June 1, 2007

Gaist, D. MD PhD, Jeppesen, U. MD PhD, Andersen, M. MD PhD, García Rodríguez, L. A., MD MSc, Hallas, J. MD PhD and Sindrup, S. H, MD PhD, "Statins and risk of polyneuropathy: A case-control study", *Neurology May 14, 2002 vol. 58 no. 9 1333-1337*

Gamelin, L., Boisdron-Celle, M., Delva, R., Geurin-Meyer, V., Ifrah, N., Morel, A., et al. "Prevention of Oxaliplatin-Related Neurotoxicity by Calcium and Magnesium Infusions: A Retrospective Study of 161 Patients Receiving Oxaliplatin Combined With 5-Fluourouracil and Leucovorin for Advanced Colorectal Cancer. *Clinical Cancer Research* 10(12, pt. 1) (2004): 4055–4061.

Goldstein D. J., et al. Duloxetine vs. Placebo in Patients with Painful Diabetic Neuropathy. *Pain* 116 (2005): 109–18.

Goldstein, M. R., Mascitelli, L., Pezzetta, F. "Do Statins Prevent or Promote Cancer?" *Curr. Oncol.* 15(2) (April 2008): 76–77.

Golomb, B. A., et al. (2007) "Physician Response to Patient Reports of Adverse Drug Effects: Implications for Patient-Targeted Adverse Effect Surveillance." *Drug Safety.* 30(8) (2007): 669-675.

Goransson, L. G., Tjensvoll, A. B., Herigstad, A., Mellgren, S. I., Omdal, R. "Small-Diameter Nerve Fiber Neuropathy in Systemic Lupus Erythematosus." *Arch. Neurol.* 63 (2006): 401–404.

Gregg, E. W., Gu, Q., Williams, D., et al. "Prevalence of Lower Extremity Diseases Associated With Normal Glucose Levels, Impaired Fasting Glucose, and Diabetes Among US Adults Aged 40 or Older." *Diabetes Res. Clin. Pract.* 77 (2007): 485–488.

Grogan, P. M.; Katz, J. S. "Toxic Neuropathies." *Neurol. Clin.* 23, (2005): 377–396.

Hammack, J., Michalak, J., Loprinzi, C., Sloan, J., Novotny, P., Soori, G., et al. "Phase III Evaluation of Nortriptyline for Alleviation of Symptoms of Cis-Platinum–Induced Peripheral Neuropathy." *Pain* 98(1–2) (2002): 195–203.

Hilpert, F., Stahle, A., Tome, O., Burges, A., Rossner, D., Spatke, K., et al. "Neuroprotection With Amifostine in the First-Line Treatment of Advanced Ovarian Cancer With Carboplatin/Paclitaxel-Based Chemotherapy—A Double-Blind, Placebo-Controlled, Randomized Phase II Study From the Arbeitsgemeinschaft Gynäkologische Onkologoie (AGO) Ovarian Cancer Study Group. *Supportive Care in Cancer* 13(10) (2005): 797–805.

Hsieh, S. T., Lin, W. "Modulation of Keratinocyte Proliferation by Skin Innervation." *J. Invest. Dermatol.* 113 (1999): 579–586.

Jacob, S., Henriksen, E. J., Schiemann, A. L., et al. "Enhancement of Glucose Disposal in Patients With Type 2 Diabetes by Alpha-Lipoic Acid." *Arzneimittelforschung* 45 (1995): 872--74.

Jiang, H., Shi, K., Li, X., Zhou, W., & Cao, Y. "Clinical Study on the Wrist-Ankle Acupuncture Treatment for 30 Cases of Diabetic Peripheral Neuritis." *Journal of Traditional Chinese Medicine* 26(1) (2006): 8–12.

King, D. S., Wilburn, A. J., Wofford, M. R., Harrell, T. K., Lindley, B. J., Jones, D. W. (2003) "Cognitive Impairment Associated With Atorvastatin and Simvastatin. *Pharmacotherapy* 23(12) (2003):1663–7.

Kwang, K. K., et al. (2008). "Simvastatin Improves Flow-Mediated Dilation but Reduces Adiponectin Levels and Insulin Sensitivity in Hypercholesterolemic Patient." *Diabetes* 31 (2008): 776–782.

Lacomis, D. "Small Fiber Neuropathy." *Muscle Nerve* 26 (2002): 173–188.

Larson AM, Polson J, Fontana RJ, Davern TJ, Lalani E, Hynan LS, Reisch JS, Schiødt FV, Ostapowicz G, Shakil AO, Lee WM; Acute Liver Failure Study Group.

"Acetaminophen-induced acute liver failure: results of a United States multicenter, prospective study". *Hepatology.* 2005 Dec;42(6):1364-72

Lazarou, J., Pomeranz, B. H., Corey, P. N. "Incidence of Adverse Drug Reactions in Hospitalized Patients: A Meta-Analysis of Prospective Studies." *JAMA* 279(15) (April 1998): 1200–5.

Lee, J. L., Low, J. A., Croakin, E., Parks, R., Berman, A. W., Mannan, N. et al. "Changes in Neurologic Function Tests May Predict Neurotoxicity Caused by Ixabepilone." *Journal of Clinical Oncology* 24(13) (2006): 2084-2091.

Lees, G., & Leach, M. J. (1993). "Studies on the Mechanism of Action of the Novel Anticonvulsant Lamotrigine (Lamictal) Using Primary Neurological Cultures From Rat Cortex." *Brain Research* 612 (1993): 190–199.

Leonard, D. R., Farooqi, M. H., & Myers, S. "Restoration of Sensation, Reduced Pain, and Improved Balance in Subjects With Diabetic Peripheral Neuropathy." *Diabetes Care* 27(1) (2004): 168–172.

Lindeman, E., Leffers, P., Spaans, F., Drukker, J., Kerckhoffs, M., & Koke, A. "Strength Training in Patients With Myotonic Dystrophy and Hereditary Motor and Sensory Neuropathy: A Randomized Clinical Trial." *Archives of Physical Medicine and Rehabilitation* 76(7) (1995): 612–620.

Maestri, A., De Pasquale Ceratti, A., Cundari, S., Zanna, C., Cortesi, E., & Crino, L. "A Pilot Study on the Effect of Acetyl-L-Carnitine in Paclitaxel- and Cisplatin-Induced Peripheral Neuropathy." *Tumori* 91(2) (2005): 135–138.

Mahley, R. W., K. H. Weisgraber, and T. P. Bersot. "Disorders of Lipid Metabolism." In *Williams Textbook of Endocrinology*, edited by H. M. Kronenberg, S. Melmed, K. S. Polonsky and P. R. Larsen. Philadelphia, PA: Saunders, Elsevier, 2008.

Marrs, J., & Newton, S. (2003). "Updating Your Peripheral Neuropathy Know-How." *Clinical Journal of Oncology Nursing* 7(3) (2003): 299–303.

Merriam-Webster's Collegiate Dictionary, 11th edition.

Meydani, M., "Vitamin E," *Lancet* 345 (January 21, 1995): 170–75.

Mizisin, A. P.; Powell, H. C. "Toxic Neuropathies." *Curr. Opin. Neuro.* 8 (1995): 367-371.

Moore, D., Donnelly, J., McGuire, W. P., Almadrones, L., Cella, D. F., Herzog, T. J., et al. "Limited Access Trial Using Amifostine for Protection Against Cisplatin and Three-Hour Paclitaxel-Induced Neurotoxicity: A Phase II Study of the Gynecologic Oncology Group." *Journal of Clinical Oncology* 21(22), (2003): 4207–4213.

Moulin D. E., et al. "Pharmacological Management of Chronic Neuropathic Pain. Consensus Statement and Guidelines From the Canadian Pain Society." *Pain Res. Manage.* 12(1) (2007): 13–21.

Novak, V., Freimer, M. L., Kissel, J. T., Sahenk, Z., Periquet, I. M., Nash, S. M., Collins, M. P., Mendell, J. R. "Autonomic Impairment in Painful Neuropathy." *Neurology* 56 (2001): 861–868.

Openshaw, H., Beamon, K., Synold, T. W., Lougmate, J., Slatkin, N. E., Doroshaw, J. H., et al. "Neurophysiological Study of Peripheral Neuropathy After High-Dose Paclitaxel: Lack of Neuroprotective Effect of Amifostine. *Clinical Cancer Research* 10(2) (2004): 461–467.

Orstavik, K., Norheim, I., Jorum, E. "Pain and Small-Fiber Neuropathy in Patients With Hypothyroidism." *Neurology* 67 (2006): 786–791.

Pace, A., Savarese, A., Picardo, M., Maresca, V., Pacetti, U., Del Monte, G., et al. "Neuroprotective Effect of Vitamin E Supplementation in Patients Treated With Cisplatin Chemotherapy." *Journal of Clinical Oncology* 21(5), (2003): 927–931.

Paice, J. A. "Peripheral Neuropathy: Experimental Findings, Clinical Approaches." *Journal of Supportive Oncology* 5(2) (2007): 61–63.

Pahor, M., Guralnik, J. M., Salive M. E., Corti, M. C., Carbonin, P., Havlik, R. J. "Do Calcium Channel Blockers Increase Risk of Cancer?" *Am. J. Hypertens.* 9(7) (July 1996): 695–9.

Phillips, K. D., Skelton, W. D., & Hand, G. A. (2004). "Effect of Acupuncture Administered in a Group Setting on Pain and Subjective Peripheral Neuropathy in Persons With Human Immunodeficiency Virus Disease." *Journal of Alternative and Complementary Medicine* 10(3) (2004): 449–455.

Pieber, K., Herceg, M., Paternostro-Sluga, T. (April 2010). "Electrotherapy for the Treatment of Painful Diabetic Peripheral Neuropathy: A Review." *J. Rehabil. Med.* 42(4): (April 2010): 289–95. doi:10.2340/16501977-0554. PMID 20461329.

Poncelet, A. N. "An Algorithm for the Evaluation of Peripheral Neuropathy." *Am. Family Physician* 57(4) (February 15, 1998): 755–764.

Postma, T. J. & Heiman, J. J. (2000). Grading of Chemotherapy-Induced Peripheral Neuropathy. *Annals of Oncology* 11 (2000): 509–513.

Preiss, D., et al. (2011). "Risk of Incident Diabetes With Intensive-Dose Compared With Moderate-Dose Statin Therapy:

A Meta-Analysis JAMA. 2011;305(24):2556-2564. doi: 10.1001/jama.2011.860

Prendergast, J. J., Miranda, G., & Sanchez, M. (2004). "Improvement of Sensory Impairment in Patients With Peripheral Neuropathy." *Endocrine Practice* 10(1), (2004): 24–30.

Puri, V., Chaudhry, N., Tatke, M., Prakash, V. "Isolated Vitamin E Deficiency With Demyelinating Neuropathy." *Muscle and Nerve* 32(2) (2005): 119-240, (8).

Rao, R. D., Flynn, P. J., Sloan, J. A., Wong, G. Y., Novotny, P., Johnson, D. B., et al. (2008). "Efficacy of Lamotrigine in the Management of Chemotherapy-Induced Peripheral Neuropathy: A phase III Randomized, Double Blind, Placebo-Controlled Trial, N01C3." *Cancer* 112(12) (2008): 2802–2808.

Ravi, R. D., Michalack, J. C., Sloan, J. A., Loprinzi, C. L., Soori, G. S., Nikcevich, D. A. et al. "Efficacy of Gabapentin in the Management of Chemotherapy-Induced Peripheral Neuropathy." *Cancer* 110 (9) (2007): 2110–2118.

Reichstein, L., Labrenz, S., Ziegler, D., & Martin, S. (2005). "Effective Treatment of Symptomatic Diabetic Polyneuropathy by High-Frequency External Muscle Stimulation." *Diabetologia* 48(5) (2005): 824–828.

Richardson, J. K., Sandman, D., & Vela, S. (2001). "A Focused Exercise Regimen Improves Clinical Measures of Balance in Patients With Peripheral Neuropathy." *Archives of Physical Medicine and Rehabilitation* 82(2) (2001): 205–209.

Rosenzweig, J. L., Ferrannini, E., Grundy, S. M., Haffner, S. M., Heine, R. J., Horton, E. S., et al. "Primary Prevention of Cardiovascular Disease and Type 2 Diabetes in Patients at Metabolic Risk: An Endocrine Society Clinical

Practice Guideline." *J. Clin. Endocrinol. Metab.* 93 (2008): 3671–3689.

Rowbotham M. C., et al. "Venlafaxine Extended Release in the Treatment of Painful Diabetic Neuropathy: A Double-Blind, Placebo-Controlled Study." *Pain* 110: (2004): 697–706. (Erratum in 2005; 113:248).

Rubin, R. et. al. "Elevated Depression Symptoms, Antidepressant Medicine Use, and Risk of Developing Diabetes During the Diabetes Prevention Program." *Diabetes Care* 31 (2008): 420–426.

Saarto, T., Wiffen, P. J. "Antidepressants for Neuropathic Pain." *Cochrane Database of Systematic Reviews 2007*, Issue 4. doi: 10.1002/14651858.CD005454.pub2.

Sen, C. K., Khanna, S., Roy, S. "Tocotrienols: Vitamin E Beyond Tocopherols." *Life Sci.* 78 (2006): 2088–98.

Shlay, J. D., Chaloner, K., Max, M. B., Flaws, B., Reichelderfer, P., Wentworth, D., et al. "Acupuncture and Amitriptyline for Pain Due to HIV-Related Peripheral Neuropathy." *JAMA* 280(18) (1998): 1590–1595.

Sindrup S. H., et al. Venlafaxine vs. "Imipramine in Painful Polyneuropathy: A Randomized, Controlled Trial." *Neurology* 60 (2003): 1284–1289.

Singleton, J. R., Smith, A. G., Brumberg, M. B. "Painful Sensory Polyneuropathy Associated With Impaired Glucose Tolerance." *Muscle Nerve* 24 (2001): 1225–1228.

Smith, A. G., Singleton, J. R. "Impaired Glucose Tolerance and Neuropathy." *Neurologist* 14 (2008): 23–29.

Smyth, J. F., Bowman, A., Perren, T., Wilkinson, P., Prescott, R. J., Quinn, K. J., et al. "Glutathione Reduces the Toxicity and Improves Quality of Life of Women Diagnosed With Ovarian Cancer Treated With Cisplatin: Results of a

Double-Blind, Randomized Trial." *Annals of Oncology* 8(6) (1997): 569–573.

Bangalore, S., Parkar, S., Grossman E., Messerli, F. H. "A Meta-Analysis of 94,492 Patients With Hypertension Treated With Beta Blockers to Determine the Risk of New-Onset Diabetes Mellitus." *Am. J. Cardiol.* 100 (8) (2007): 1254–1262.

Stafford, R. S. "Regulating Off-Label Drug Use — Rethinking the Role of the FDA." *New England Journal of Medicine* 358 (2008): 1427–1429.

Strauss, M. H. and Hall, A. S. "Angiotensin Receptor Blockers May Increase Risk of Myocardial Infarction: Unraveling the ARB-MI Paradox." *Am. J. Circulation* 114 (2006): 838–854.

Streeper, R. S., Henriksen, E. J., Jacob, S., et al. "Differential Effects of Lipoic Acid Stereoisomers on Glucose Metabolism in Insulin-Resistant Skeletal Muscle." *Am. J. Physiol.* 273 (1997): E185–E191.

Stubblefield, M. D., Vahdat, L. T., Balmaceda, C. M., Troxel, A. B., Hesdorffer, C. S., & Gooch, C. L. "Glutamine as a Neuroprotective Agent in High-Dose Paclitaxel-Induced Peripheral Neuropathy: A Clinical and Electrophysiologic Study." *Clinical Oncology* 17(4), (2005): 71–276.

Tanyel, M. C., Mancano, L. D. "Neurologic Findings in Vitamin E Deficiency." *Am. Fam. Physician* 55 (1997): 197–201. [PubMed abstract]

Traber, M. G. "Vitamin E Regulatory Mechanisms." *Annu. Rev. Nutr.* 27 (2007): 347–62.

Traber, M. G. "Vitamin E." In *Modern Nutrition in Health and Disease*, edited by M. E. Shils, M. Shike, A. C. Ross, B. Caballero and R. Cousins, 396-411. Baltimore, MD: Lippincott, Williams & Wilkins, 2006.

Tütüncü, N. B., Bayraktar, M. and Varli, K. "Reversal of Defective Nerve Conduction With Vitamin E Supplementation in Type 2 Diabetes: A Preliminary Study." *Diabetes Care* 21(11) (1998): 1915–1918.

US National Library of Medicine & National Institutes of Health. Medline Plus Medical Dictionary (2003). Retrieved March 21, 2007 from http://www.nlm.nih.gov/medlineplus/mplusdictionary.html.

Vahdat, L., Papadopoulos, K., Lange, D., Leuin, S., Kaufman, E., Donovan, D., et al. (2001). "Reduction of Paclitaxel-Induced Peripheral Neuropathy With Glutamine." *Clinical Cancer Research* 7(5) (2001): 1192–1197.

Vahidnia, A., van der Voet, G. B., de Wolff, F. A. "Arsenic Neurotoxicity—A Review." *Hum. Exp. Toxicol.* 26, (2007): 823–832.

Verhagen, H., Buijsse, B., Jansen, E., Bueno-de-Mesquita, B. "The State of Antioxidant Affairs." *Nutr. Today* 41 (2006): 244–50.

Von Delius, S., Eckel, F., Wagenpfeil, S., Mayr, M., Stock, K., Kullmann, F., et al. (2007). "Carbamazepine for prevention of oxaliplatin-related neurotoxicity in patients with advanced colorectal cancer: Final results of a randomized, controlled, multicenter phase II study." *Investigational New Drugs* 25(2) (2007): 173–180.

Wagstaff, L. R., Mitton, M. W., Arvik, B. M., Doraiswamy, P. M. "Statin-Associated Memory Loss: Analysis of 60 Case Reports and Review of the Literature." *Pharmacotherapy* 23(7) (July 2003): 871-80.

Wang, W., Lin, J., Lin, T., Chen, W., Jiang, J., Wang, H., et al. "Oral Glutamine is Effective for Preventing Oxaliplatin-Induced Neuropathy in Colorectal Cancer Patients." *Oncologist* 12(3) (2007): 312–319.

Weimer L. H., "Medication-Induced Peripheral Neuropathy". *Curr. Neurol. Neurosci. Rep.* (Jan 2003).

White, C. M., Pritchard, J., & Turner-Stokes, L. "Exercise for People with Peripheral Neuropathy." *Cochrane Database of Systematic Reviews 2004*, Issue 4. doi:10.1002/14651858.CD003904.pub2.

Wiffen, P. J., et al. "Gabapentin for Acute and Chronic Pain." *Cochrane Database of Syst. Rev.* (3) (2005):CD005452.

Wilkes, G. M. & Barton-Burke, M. (2005). *2005 Oncology Nursing Drug Handbook*, Sudbury, MA: Jones & Bartlett.

Wilkes, G. "Peripheral Neuropathy Related to Chemotherapy." *Seminars in Oncology Nursing* 23(3) (2007): 162–73. doi:10.1016/j.soncn.2007.05.001. PMID 17693343.

Wong, R., & Sagar, S. (2006). "Acupuncture Treatment for chemotherapy-induced peripheral neuropathy—A case series." *Acupuncture in Medicine* 24(2) (2006): 87–91.

Ziegler, D., Nowak, H., Kempler, P., Vargha, P., & Low, P. A. "Treatment of Symptomatic Diabetic Polyneuropathy with the Antioxidant Alpha-Lipoic Acid: A Meta-Analysis." *Diabetic Medicine* 21(2) (2004): 114–121.

Zivkovic, S., Lacomis, D., Guiliani, M., "Sensory Neuropathy Associated With Metronidazole: Report of Four Cases and Review of the Literature." *J. Clinical Neuromuscular Disease* 3 (2001): 8–12.

Made in the USA
Lexington, KY
30 June 2015